The Thirteen-Hour Life Coach

Simon Arnold

This book is dedicated to my two sons, Aston and Ayden.
May you both live long and very successful lives.

Contents

Introduction - The Thirteen-Hour Life Coach

In April 2020, I moved from Berlin to Bayern in Germany and spent a few days registering myself and my kids with new doctors. During my youngest son's initial assessment, the doctor asked me a few questions as to where I come from and how I landed in Bayern. I told her I had been recently diagnosed with Attention Deficit Hyperactivity Disorder (ADHD) and that living in the mountains would be better for me. I showed her the notes I was currently writing on the subject and she wanted to know more. I explained I was writing about *success strategies for adults with ADHD.*

She immediately said that the text books she had on the subject where quite old and promoted more of the negative aspects of the disorder. She thought a positive view would be great and suggested I write a book about it. I told her it would be in English and she said she would take an English copy of the book as soon as possible, indicating a desperate need for something different, new and exciting about this condition.

I left the practice surprised.

Over the next two days, I registered with more doctors and they asked me similar questions. They too thought writing a book would be a great idea, and would want a copy.

Up until now, I had been writing notes to make my life easier. I didn't know what I was doing could benefit other people. So, I started the book, working on it for 2 hours a day. It took some getting used to.

I had been taking medication for ADHD since my diagnosis in December 2019, had a new personality, was hyper-focusing on what was in front of me instead of being aware of my surroundings and felt I was living two separate lives. Fortunately, I had written a diary every day since 2006, so for 15 years I had a blueprint to my life. I just knew that I could solve all of the problems I was having and *fast!*

I knew if I was having major problems, *others* must be too.

Before I knew it, I was up to 200 hours of writing. It was therapeutic! I bought 50 A4 note pads and loads of pens and highlighters from a discount store and wrote down everything that came into my mind about the condition, but the problems I was having with the disorder were immense!

I couldn't do this alone: I reached out to a brilliant psychiatrist but he was falling way too short. I needed more help, more assistance, but I couldn't find it. So, I decided that I would take on this dilemma myself.

I live in two mazes every day. One of distraction and one of total clarity. I wanted to know each maze intimately. I had to see this as a game. I could do it!

I took every negative message from my diaries, analysed them and, where possible, put a positive spin on them! And I would get help in my daily life too. A neighbour gave me pointers in how I could socialise better, this spurred me on to write Chapter Nine.

But, after a few months of writing, I was getting really tired. I would be solidifying ideas from people I met and getting help from my inner voice, which, before using medication for ADHD, I had never experienced before. I kept writing every single day. And then, after 400 hours into the book, I couldn't do anything right. I was at a plateau. I was really stuck. I had nothing else to go on.

I sat poised to write the 401st hour looking at the 22 self-help books on my desk knowing that none of them could help me at that moment.

So, I changed tack.

I decided to use the success strategies I had written about ADHD into practice. They worked. I was so impressed I decided to launch an ADHD success group in my local town. I had found solutions which increased the value of my life. Everyone with ADHD had to know about this! I launched the ADHD success group on the meet-up website in September 2020 and realised that the book had to be finished. I had to get the information out to more people.

After 730 hours, I finished this book.

This book changes the status quo!

If you have ADHD, or believe you could have it, his book is written for you.

I hope you enjoy it.

How to use this book
This book offers a fresh perspective on living a successful life with attention deficit hyperactivity disorder (ADHD) and for those that think they have it.
Each chapter gives the reader an insight into what living with ADHD is like and details the most important part of each with a principles section, acting as a summary.
First, read through the book in it's entirety. Then, choose sections which are most relevant to your life, that is, relationships or socialising, look at the principles and work them.

Chapter One – The life coach

This morning, I woke up as Simon and within one hour some other guy just turns up, orders my life for 13 hours and disappears in the night.

I met him for the first time in March 2020. He crept up on me slowly while I was filing paperwork at home. Instead of haphazardly shoving documents into a folder, I ordered them in a neat and orderly manner.

'This isn't normal,' I thought.

I switched on a reading light and there was silence.

The sound of the clock, the birds outside, even the humming of the radiator were all passive.

'Why is everything still?' I thought to myself, looking at my hands and legs.

I grabbed a book, opening it to the first chapter and read the first few pages. The words seemed to jump out at me. It was weird. After ten minutes I put it down, grab my mobile phone and call my wife.

She asked what I was doing.

'Reading' I said.

'What are you reading?', she asked.

I told her the name of the book, the author and a summary of what I had just read.

'That sounds good' she replied. 'You can't usually tell me the author, let alone go into details.'

'It *is* normal to read a novel three or four times through before you understand it, right?' I asked enquiringly, while holding and turning the book in my hands.

'Of course not!' she replied. 'Perhaps a text book, but a novel you understand on the first read. That's the idea.'

'Wait a minute' I said, holding the first Harry Potter book in my hand. 'I couldn't remember the characters of Harry Potter, apart from Harry, even though I read the first three books three times through, remember that!'

'I have just understood a whole chapter of a book.'

I stopped, put the book down and looked around the room for an explanation.

'Are you okay?', my wife asked.

'I am okay but also not okay,' I answered, standing up from my chair while laughing and crying at the same time.

'*I can understand what I read!*' I shouted.

'Does that mean I can understand the letters I get in the post?' I say enthusiastically.

'Probably,' she said, wondering where I was going with this.

'You have always read them to me. What if *that* has changed?!'

'I think you are getting a little ahead of yourself,' my wife said.

'See you tonight' she said putting down the phone.

I stood up, not knowing what was happening. I felt whole.

'Where have you come from?' I said out loud, standing limp with tears running down my face.

'I have always been here,' came the reply.

I look around startled this time.

'Don't worry' said a voice 'No one is here except yourself.'

I stayed steadfast.

'*I'm your organised self,*' the voice replied soothingly.

My eyes slowly scan the room randomly trying to process what I thought I had just heard. I was thinking someone was outside. No one was there when I looked.

'I'm here for most of the day today.' the soft voice whispered, as I retreat from my office window.

'And why not, all of the day?' I asked in a shallow and slow voice sitting back down in the chair.

'For thirteen hours a day for the rest of your life, I will be here,' came the reply.

The voice was gone.

'Thirteen exact hours and no longer?' I contemplated to myself.

I thought if this voice, guy or whatever it was came back tomorrow then I won't miss the opportunity. Instead, I will take it.

Principle

– Accept the changes that life hands you.

Chapter Two – Big Mo

The next day the voice appeared again. Naming it the 'voice' would be creepy and stupid so I chose Big Mo. *Big* for being the cool voice and *Mo* for the moments he is here.

I wanted to share the feeling of reading and understanding a book for the first time with everyone but decided to keep it under wraps. I knew something had changed but didn't know the specifics.

Big Mo asked me if I have ever heard my inner voice. I admitted that I hadn't.

He explained that the inner voice first appears when a child is seven years old. An American psychiatrist called Dr Russell A. Barkley describes this as the *mind's voice*.

'The book you read and understood yesterday for the *first time* has something to do with the inner voice. Except your brain didn't develop in a normal manner. From what I can make out, there is a delay in certain signals being sent to the correct part of your brain at the required time'. These signals help with something called your 'executive function' finished Mo.

'Normal adults with a good functioning brain can, according to Dr Barkley, "… hold in mind what we have silently read to ourselves." (2010: 78)

'You are just finding this out now!'

'So, my brain works like a normal person's brain?' I asked Mo.

'Exactly' said Mo. 'A normal functioning human brain is called neurotypical.'

'So, you are saying the connections in my brain are wired correctly and the signals are reaching where they need to go?' I asked.

'Yes, you can now converse with your core self.' he continued.

'This is your second chance. Make the most of the thirteen hours we have together and don't worry when I come later to you in the morning or leave earlier in the evening than you expected'.

Principle

– The mind's voice will be your best guide in life. Listen to it!

Chapter Three – A new working memory

I realised I had a new working memory and needed to start slow.

One day, I picked three books to read with my youngest son. The pictures were now gleaming with action and the text was really funny. But I chose the wrong time to read to him, so decided to alter my daily routine.

I get up early to revel in the peace and quiet of a new day.

If you have a comfortable place to sit, put on a light and read. I feel the sun's rays coming through the window lighting up the room. Living in a valley gives me a chance to watch the local mountain slowly turn into colour with a cup of herbal tea in my hand. What would you notice when you get up early?

When my youngest awakes, we read without distraction.

I put on the radio a little later on, which I love so much more now.

'With a big smile on your face,' said Big Mo.

'It was you who made me see radio and music in a different way,' I said.

'How can people put the radio on and not be disturbed by it?' I said out loud as my wife entered the kitchen.

'Because it's background music!' she said switching on the coffee machine.

Filtering my environment for the first time was exciting!

Up until now *all* sounds were in my foreground. Everything was competing for my attention. Can you get what I mean?

'This is when music turns into a luxury item,' Big Mo said.

'A song you have heard a thousand times is more alive, you hear the lyrics and sense the feelings and hidden messages. It is similar to skipping the words in a book but instead of hearing a couple of words and then noise and a couple of words again the music runs smoothly now.'

But I knew I heard the radio in a new way. It was a novelty. I thought I should just listen to the news snippet for a couple of minutes and then turn it off. That would suffice.

As my family sit down for breakfast at the dining table, I move a box containing a fidget spinner, a tangle wild toy, a snow globe and a wooden 3D puzzle of a small town to its edge. These items keep the kids busy and on their bottoms. Each place mat is set the night before.

The canter of the table is waved as well as the bench we sit on to occupy fidgety hands.

'You don't get annoyed with your kids like you did before,' said Mo.

'I guess I have an extra second to think about a situation before responding to it,' I replied.

'I was trying to lead by example but it was really difficult to pack the kids school bags with exercise books, a homework folder, drink and food. It was always way too much for me!'

'If you didn't see normal you didn't see what it takes to be a *leader*,' said Big Mo.

'But this is what I have to be when I have two children of school age. There is just no other way,' I said answering him.

I knew I had difficulties. My wife and I would complete set routines or jobs but I knew that I was the one falling behind, not her. She even organised me! Does that seem familiar in your life?

'Why?' asked Mo.

Because I couldn't make head nor tail of even small organisational matters that arose. This is due to the difficulties in the four areas of thinking that affect people with Attention Deficit Hyperactivity Disorder (ADHD). These are 'nonverbal working memory, verbal working memory, emotion regulation and planning/problem solving'. (Barkley, 2010: 69).

Dr Russell A. Barkley suggests "As an adult with ADHD, you've been subjected to delayed development of each of the four executive functions." (2010: 71)

'That's one reason why you get your wife to help with the kids' homework,' said Mo.

'Yes. After school she reads the homework and messages and completes with them what is due for the next day. If I have to do it, I get really nervous!'

'It is only homework!' said Mo.

'I could never read or understand homework for 42 years.' I replied disappointed.

'It is their homework, not yours. It's them, not you,' said Mo.

'And when they get rowdy and don't want to do it? What then?' I ask Mo.

'Think about what author and pastor John Maxwell wrote in his book *What Successful People Know About Leadership*.'

"Treat them not as they are, but as they could be." (Maxwell, 2016: 142)

You could try this too!

In the evening, we eat supper together, the living room is quite a mess at the end of a busy day so I remind the kids, occasionally, of a conversation I had with a 90-year-old pub owner I worked for in my twenties. She said 'When you go from one room to another Simon, please take something that needs to be moved with you'. I never forgot this advice, probably because she knew I wasn't doing this. Now with forethought I can do this more easily.

When the things are in their rightful place the kids can play pool or with their toys.

They then listen to a story on their smart speakers before bedtime until they fall asleep.

'You then slowly leave me for the day' I said to Big Mo with a lump in my throat.

It took a while to know when this would happen, but now I can time it well.

Until recently, I was just overwhelmed by my environment. Mo has taken this uncomfortable feeling away so every night I take a moment to appreciate how my life has changed – to love both versions of myself.

When everyone is asleep, I walk around my home. Each picture on the wall contains stories influenced by undiagnosed ADHD and fear of my environment. I know that the pictures I put up in the future will be ones containing narratives of joy.

As I lay myself down on my bed one night Mo said to me

'It is now time to embrace life fully.'

'I thought you had gone for the night.' I said with a smile.

'How about we visit a local *bewirtschaftet* hut in your area tomorrow?'

'Sounds like a great idea,' I replied.

Principles

- Wake up early to the peace and quiet of a new day.
- Read books with a positive or funny message to yourself or to your children. Your new interest will keep them motivated too.
- Listen to the news snippet on the radio and then turn it off.
- Wooden toys and hand-held fun games (no electronics) are great. Have 'touch specific' regions – a curvy bench or table with interesting features to occupy fidgety hands.
- Take an extra second to think about a situation before responding to it.
- Pack the kids' school bags or your work bag the night before. Prepare food and drink to take in the morning.
- Dr Russell A. Barkley: "As an adult with ADHD, you've been subjected to delayed development of each of the four executive functions." (2010: 71) At least you know. This book is here to support you!
- Ask for help. We all have strengths and weaknesses. Concentrate on your strengths.
- On children – John Maxwell, "Treat them not as they are, but as they could be."
- Place emphasis on taking things to their rightful place before the end of the day.
- Games such as pool, kicker and board games are socially healthy.

Chapter Four – The hut

'The piece of conglomerate in my hand looks like nails have been hammered so hard into the rock that just the head is visible', I say to myself sitting in a local alpine hut inspecting what I am looking at.

I live in the most southern region of Germany called the Allgäu, home of the Nagelfluhkette, a nature reserve with these strange rocks found at the edge of the Alpine region.

I sat there wondering how I was going to lead my new life.

I had heard that ADHD affects everything I do and the way I think. I also live in a different country to which I grew up in, so there were many aspects I wanted to understand.

'Which is where we start today!' said Big Mo surprising me as I drink my tea.

'That would be great,' I said.

'How are you feeling?' asked Mo.

'I feel good because so many distractions have disappeared from my life,' looking around me watching the hut filling up with more people.

'I would like to know if my own Englishness is holding me back here in Germany, before we discuss ADHD, if you don't mind.'

'No problem' said Mo easing into the mindful conversation.

'You were bought up with different values, perceptions and culture to what you have now but you have assimilated to this country – You have grown.' Mo said.

'Thanks,' I replied.

The tone of the German language is very monotonous. Dialects and personal traits raise the volume and pitch which at first you tended to believe people are having a go at each other, when in fact they are having a conversation.

'But as you learnt from the speaker Les Brown, 'death and life are in the tongue.'

'Yes, I had to get this right as quick as possible,' I said.

'But you could only do this by conducting yourself according to others when you started to live in Germany. I remember a time you were at a party, a few months after arriving, you were having fun but the host told you a few times to just speak German.'

'I was trying to relax and enjoy myself,' I said.

'It wasn't that you weren't speaking German, because you were, you just weren't fluent enough by then,' said Mo. 'She was right in encouraging you to speak German, but I think as the years went on in this country people were still dishing out "what you should be doing" and you were getting fed up with it.'

'I guess after a while I could speak fluent German but found that while I was working on myself not many others were,' I said.

'And you saw that!' said Mo. 'I don't think you necessarily have your Englishness holding you back I think, but instead, the motivation to learn knowing that others are giving you inaccurate advice after a while is where you differ!'

'But, on the other hand, you have lived here for eleven years and should be well up to speed but you aren't. I also think that you are edge because you don't hear your own language around you anymore,.'

'You are right,' I said.

'Listen (said Mo). I am the one in your head so I need to settle you down to settle the part of me down, if you know what I am saying?'

'You have to remember that to a certain extent people can assimilate to a country but a big chunk of ourselves or conditioning won't go away and is something you should be comfortable with. This doesn't concern anyone else!' Mo said.

'But the biggest issue is ADHD,' he finished.

'Okay,' I said.

'Interaction with the outside world has to be done differently now,' he said.

'What do you suggest?' I asked him.

'Start following the advice from Dr Russell Barkley about self-control! He says, "Self-control is a *self-directed* action. This means instead of acting in direct response *toward* an event, you stop and take action toward yourself".' (2010: 65)

'Do you mean stopping to pause?' I asked.

'That is exactly what I mean,' said Mo.

'But don't neurotypical people have trouble saying something without thinking it through?' I asked.

'Yes, of course, but you have always been impulsive and blurted something out.' said Mo.

'So, I guess I can give myself space to breathe when I hadn't before?' I said.

'Yes, definitely,' he said suggesting that I pause quickly now and take a sip of the hot ginger and honey tea that is standing on the table.

'But people will see less of a reaction and think something is wrong!' I exclaim.

'Not necessarily!' said Mo.

'Remember, just because you know you have ADHD other people won't. It is a normal human reaction to stop and consider what is said before answering.'

'But how can I stop making too many mistakes!' I said blurting out. I'm always apologising to people because I have never been up to speed,' I said.

'Look, it is difficult having me in your head. You have to get used to it,' replied Mo.

'You have the willingness to say that you made a mistake but you can learn from these mistakes *now*!'

'How come?' I ask.

'Because you have a good functioning brain.'

'It just all seems a bit too much,' I said.

'I get it,' said Mo 'Then try something I came up with yesterday that extends the time frame of a certain situation. I call it "courteous caving in".'

'What is that?' I asked.

'"Courteous caving in" is about giving yourself time to be on your own to calm down and think!' finished Mo.

'Is that meant to be a joke?' I said scorning him.

'No, it isn't. You will feel that you need more insight into a particular situation or life event. Be kind to yourself, search out a quiet place and think things through. You will have to learn from your experiences and to know when to stay quiet.'

'And if I cannot retreat from a situation, what then?,' I asked.

'Then just keep your poise, breathe and try to answer accordingly.'

We sat for a while longer together in the alpine hut.

Mo didn't appear for the whole of the afternoon but as I was settling down to sleep at night, he whispered something in my ear which comforted me.

'If you go through life wanting to fit in and you haven't, you just haven't yet found out what you are meant to do in this lifetime.'

I smiled. I knew what the next assignment was!

Principles

- Living close to nature gives your life serenity.
- Not knowing how to live life with ADHD is totally normal. ADHD affects everything you do and the way you think. This is why this book has been written!

- Not hearing your own language spoken in a foreign country can make you 'on-edge'. This is normal.
- Again, think first before you react!
- Just because you know you have ADHD other people won't.
- Be willing to admit mistakes and to learn from them.
- *Courteous caving in.* Knowing you need more insight into a particular situation or life event. Be kind to yourself, search out a quiet place and think things through.
- You don't need to fit in with everyone.

Chapter Five – A different spin on change

Having a new working memory comes without a personal instruction manual.

I knew I could adapt to life's challenges but this time I guessed I could really make a mark.

So I bought a huge whiteboard and stood it in my bedroom. I wrote down five goals to concentrate on, which would take my focus off the ADHD.

I got the idea from Russell Barkley who states that people with ADHD have an "…incredible capacity for goal-directed creativity, innovation and problem solving." And that "Not only do *you* decide what to do, but you do it in a way that might not have occurred to anyone else." (2010: 87)

'You wanted to see if he was right!' said Mo.

'Yeah, I did. Dealing with ADHD in the early days was a real shit storm, I had no one to ask what I was going through and no one could emphasise with me. This goal setting idea was fun and if I could achieve these goals, it would mean I had basically mastered ADHD.'

I knew I needed the help of others to reach these goals but didn't have a clue how to interact properly with other people.

Mo asked me to re-read a book I had bought a few years back called *The Culture Map* by the author Erin Meyer (2014). I had used this book in the past to decode the differences in a working environment between the English and Germans and it did work. My favourite quotations from the book are "…*frame your behaviour in cultural terms*" (2014: 81) and "…in a German environment she didn't realize that being persuasive would require a different approach." (2014: 89)

'But you were trying this approach,' said Mo.

'I was trying, Erin's book is spot on, but I wasn't effective.'

'So in which area did you start with now?' asked Mo.

'I wanted to know my wife inside out!' I said.

Mo laughed hard and heartily.

'Why are you laughing?' I said.

'I wasn't expecting that' he replied, 'But it is a good start!'

'If I can do that first then I can understand other people.' I concluded.

My wife is German and I am English. I just feel that the Germans like to have all of their ideas together before they make a decision. I make a decision at the drop of a hat. I also seem to feel everything around me.

For example, I cherish the colour of the mountain trees in summer, the black squirrels that run around us while out hiking or the fresh powdered snow that fell overnight. I have naturally expected my wife to agree or show enthusiasm. But her answer, if she gave one at all, never seemed to be in tune with the gratefulness I was expressing. This always stopped me in my tracks. I didn't want her to be me, I just expected to hear a positive response as an English person would. Then I found out why this didn't happen. Kate Fox, author and anthropologist wrote in her book *Watching the English*, "…etiquette also requires that the response express agreement, as in 'Yes, isn't it?' or 'Mmm, very cold'." (2004: 28/29)

I was always expecting, as Kate suggested, '…a social *response*, not a rational answer…'(2004: 29)

My wife does appreciate her environment but because of *her* culture she is different.

'That doesn't seem that important, Simon,' replied Mo.

'It is of utmost importance' I said.

Understanding this very basic social standing meant I could then concentrate on self-control. I never realised that such small intricate language behaviour, which is different to my upbringing, could leave me so wide open.

'Do you remember my wife and I had a disagreement over a name of a mountain peak?

'Yes' said Mo. The two of you had a full-scale argument!

'The name of a mountain peak isn't a big deal,' said Mo, almost huffing.

'I guess it was to me,' I replied. I should have stayed quiet but I wanted to win the conversation. I felt my wife wanted to win also. We found out there are two mountains in the area with the same name! Except this argument wasn't healthy for either of us.

I was learning how to read social clues and how to act in certain situations.

'You couldn't access past experiences in your head to help you in your present situation, which affects your future,' Mo suggested.

'But you know what is really interesting about ADHD, which I am sure many people with the condition can appreciate,' I said.

'What's that then?' said Mo.

'If you are around people you don't know, it is easier to use self-control to not react to a situation.'

'Because they don't know you?' said Mo.

'Exactly. I have been married for fourteen years. When not reacting comes into play my wife will know that something is off. And because it is off, she says I am probably in a mood.'

'But you are just being quiet; you are not in a mood,' said Mo.

'That's what I'm trying to get across,' I answer.

There is no practice period for not saying anything.

'That's stressful for both parties,' said Mo.

'It really is,' I finish.

Do you see this in your life?

'I guess people have to live with the person you have become,' said Mo. 'Did you know it took you only three months to decide what to react to?'

'Is that good?' I asked.

'It isn't bad,' he replied

'I feel you enjoy the brain pause that neurotypical people find natural now,' said Mo.

'Which opened up a new world for you. Do you remember the day you were discussing the name of the mountain peak?'

'Of course,' I replied.

'It was really the first time you looked into your wife's eyes. I'll never forget it,' said Mo.

'Oh my God Mo, you are right,' I said. 'I never looked people in the eyes. Instead, I used my ears to understand them while looking away. My brain was blocking out the sense of sight on purpose so I wouldn't be overloaded.

'I first knew I acted this way when I was a sales assistant in a shop in Berlin. I was talking with a customer about a product for about ten minutes. When I had finished talking the lady went silent!'

'Wasn't that the example of the longest pause anyone has given you ever?' laughed Mo.

'It definitely was strange. The customer stood there looking at me in the eyes for about a minute not saying anything. I didn't know what was about to happen, to be honest. After a minute she broke eye contact. Then she spoke.'

'What did she say?' asked Mo.

'She thought at first I was completely disrespecting her. She knew I wasn't holding eye contact but became more interested in my form of communication *because* I never looked at her.'

'I don't follow you,' said Mo.

'She wanted to hear me out.'

'And then what did she say?' asked Mo.

'She complemented me,' I replied, half laughing.

'Why was that?' asked Mo.

She said 'I have never met anyone who has listened with 100% accuracy in regards to the product, the price and recommendation you gave to me on an item, without looking me in the face. I really thought you weren't being serious!'

'Did she buy the product?' asked Mo.

'She did, and she was really happy! But she did tell me that looking at someone when I was talking to them is very important.'

'But you never realised your life could be at such extremes!' said Mo.

'Why would I?' I replied. 'That was normal for me!'

'It wasn't until I was diagnosed with ADHD and medicated that I saw this strange phenomenon.'

'How did you work out in your head, these extreme life situations?' asked Mo.

'I have written a diary since 2006 and to understand myself better I have recently read through each page of the twelve books, looking at every instance in detail.'

'I guess I wrote about this customer in the hope I would one day know why the situation was so strange! But then the penny dropped!'

'It goes further?' asked Mo.

'Yeah, it does. I worked with a colleague in the same store who didn't look at me either when we were having a conversation. Other colleagues would find it hilarious how we would speak intensely with each other but look over each other's shoulders or in an entirely different direction but still find each other interesting.'

'But you realise this now because you have a completely different perspective,'

'Sounds crazy, right. But it's true.'

'I guess because the chemistry was right and the topic of conversation was working between the two of us, I never knew certain things were happening,'

But these days I talk a lot less now due to a change of personality. I know my bubbling enthusiasm is still there Mo and I guess I will get it back someday!'

'This is where I come in,' said Mo. Mo reminded me that my ADHD symptoms won't disappear. I cannot get out of its way and is probably not influenced by the foods I eat.

'I was getting used to changing on the spot. It was hardening me up for something, I just didn't know what. Because I had no prior self-talk mechanism I couldn't use my past and future predictions to help me. I was failing every single day, I never remembered my failures and always lived in the present, which, in a way, was my safety net.

'I knew I was working hard; it was only the expectations from others I couldn't match.'

'But you have built up a good habit of taking bad experiences and turning them into good ones,' said Mo.

'Yeah, that's true,' I said.

'Can you remember Mr Margrove from the language school I attended? He once said something funny.'

'Vaguely,' answered Mo.

Well, Mr Margrove was the director, I had just finished the course and went to give him back two books I had borrowed. He asked me what I intended to do next. I told him I wanted to study physiotherapy. As I put two textbooks down on his desk, he turned on his heels, walked back to his desk and smiled as he sat down.

'"I'd like you to come back, to this school," he said, flicking the first few pages of one of the books while in deep thought.

'"What do you mean?" I replied.

'"Your knowledge of the German language is good enough, but you're the first person in a very long time who's has actually shown interest in the course and you're obviously someone who doesn't want to collect unemployment benefit for the rest of their lives."

'I didn't know where he was going with this.

'"You connect with people, and I want you to come back in five years' time to tell people your story."

'"Why, Sir? And why 5 years?" I asked in amazement.

'"Because I'm sure that you could bring over to the students a certain learning process that they would find motivational."

'"Ok, but why 5 years?" I repeated.

'Mr Margrove crossed his hands, sat up abruptly and announced, "10 years is too long and I retire in six."'

'That's pretty good,' said Mo.

'"But what if I don't achieve anything?" I said to Mr Margrove before leaving the room.

'"You're not the type to just not do *anything*." He said, making a point.

'"I guess I could come back," I replied. I left his room that day feeling a little odd. I passed his course, but only just! And people that 'only just' pass anything in life aren't really that special, are they? So, I didn't end up going back to hold a presentation.'

'Hold on a minute,' said Mo. 'You are totally missing the point!'

'Which is what?' I asked.

'Can you remember when you were working as a physiotherapy assistant in your local hospital in England?'

'Yes,' I replied.

'Well, what annoyed you the most?'

'That half of the patients never completed their exercises, even if I showed them countless times.'

'Did you not see a similar story in the classroom here at this school?' asked Mo.

'Well, most never did the homework,' I replied.

'But what else?' said Mo 'looking at this from the hospital environment.'

'I don't know,' I replied.

'People didn't *want* to get better.' said Mo 'They don't want to rescue themselves. You just got on with it, you have never worried about how much work something would take and you have always wanted to improve your knowledge, whether it was on the language course or in the workplace. Mr Margrove saw this motivation in you but more importantly, you can develop others more so that you could yourself.'

'Oh, I get it, now,' I replied.

'You can also problem solve quite well because of your life experience.'

'Can you remember the audiocast from American pastor, John Maxwell?' I said.

'Oh, I know what's coming,' Mo said, laughing at himself.

'That part about changing on the *Winning is an Inside Job* CD!'.

'How did it go?' he said, intensifying the situation.

'I love playing and saying this quote over again,' I said relishing in excitement.

'*Simon, tell me for the thousandth time what he said!*'

'Okay, John Maxwell said

"You will change! Life doesn't wait for people that will not change. So the question is not are you going to change, the question is are you going to be on the front end and make money off of it, and be creative because of it, and make life changes or are you going to be on the back end..."' (2011)

'Wait a minute,' said Mo pausing, 'You changed at the front end because of your natural motivation and also on the back end too because your brain functions properly now.'

'Exactly. But that's also a bit weird, don't you think!' as we both laugh together at home on our own.

Principles

- Having a new working memory comes without a personal instruction manual. This book is your guide.

- People with ADHD have an "...incredible capacity for goal-directed creativity, innovation and problem solving." says Russell Barkley. Create new life goals. This takes your mind off ADHD.

- Someone without ADHD doesn't have the capability of feeling empathy towards you. They can, however, through compassion (a distinct emotional state) hear you out.

- Get to know the closest person in your life better than before. This can be the start of realising your own self-control.

- Understand it will take practice to know when to react appropriately in social settings.

- It is easier to use self-control around people you don't know.

- Using self- control around family members means you can be quiet and not be in a mood. You will understand this, the person who you are quiet around may not.

- Enjoy the new wonder of looking into people's eyes during conversation and seeing facial expressions.

- ADHD symptoms do not disappear. You cannot get out of its way and is probably not influenced by the foods you eat.

- A change of personality can result in taking medication for ADHD. It is scary but you have your Mo to guide you. Give yourself time to get to used to the new you!

- You don't need to prove you can pass a 'course' with top grades to believe you have something special. Other people see your best qualities, which you might not be aware of.

- Many people in life don't want to get better! They don't want to rescue themselves.

- From John Maxwell, "You will change! Life, doesn't wait for people that will not change..." You can be on the 'front' end of life by being motivated to do better. If you get successful treatment, if you believe you have ADHD yourself you can improve on the 'back' end too giving you a holistic sense of worth to move forward and be more successful in life.

Chapter Six – Physiotherapy

'Physiotherapy was a blast wasn't it?'

'I'm not really sure,' said Mo. 'I was in your head, remember, but tucked away somewhere!'

We both laughed.

'I remember spending lots of my free time at a friend's private practice in England when I was about twenty years old. I would observe literally hundreds of the patients being treated.'

'This sparked off something, didn't it?' said Mo.

'It really did,' I replied. 'I decided to live physiotherapy. At that time, I was working as a fitness instructor, but I wanted to study physiotherapy and to become qualified.'

'I remember the build up to that,' said Mo laughing his head off.

'Do you?' I asked.

'Yeah, you were at home on the south coast of England when you got this off-the-wall idea,' he said.

'What do you mean, off the wall?' I asked, flustered.

'You were looking on the internet one day after you found out that Australia was the leader in the field of manual therapy techniques. These techniques were used in the private practice where you spent lots of your time and you wanted to know more.'

'Oh yes, I remember now,' I said.

'So you came across the University of Queensland website and saw they offered the course,' continued Mo 'And what did you do?'

'I found a company that offered a foundation course I had to complete in order to study at the university,' I said.

'And then you paid the course fees there and then to this company on the same day,' Mo replied.

'True.' I did.

'The best bit was seeing your mum's reaction,' Mo said.

'I can't remember that,' I said.

'She nearly fainted in front of you,' Mo replied.

'I did just jump into it, didn't I?' I said.

'That is just so typical ADHD and you!' laughed Mo.

'So the game was on. I had no idea of how to get there or where I would live, but I didn't care. I got to know a guy called Sam at work whose parents lived in Brisbane. His parents were happy to let me and my wife (who was my girlfriend back then) stay at their place until we got onto our feet.'

'You stayed with them for three months,' said Mo.

'My wife and I were very grateful,' I said. 'We moved into our own place near to the college soon afterwards. I studied A-levels during the day and organised work experience in a private physiotherapy practice for the afternoon. Once, the practice was full with the town's female hockey team. A few of us would be taping the girls' muscles while watching *The Simpsons* on television. It is so much easier to learn something when it is fun!'

'But you were always supervised,' said Mo.

'Yes, I was. I saw new physiotherapy techniques being used and could ask why we would carry out certain movements on a limb or press on a certain point of a muscle. The year came to a close but I didn't pass the A-levels to get into the university. I had no choice but to go back to England.'

'But you picked yourself up again!' said Mo.

'True,' I replied. 'I got a job as a physiotherapy assistant at a local hospital, meanwhile applying to loads of Universities. I even paid a life coach to get me up to speed with interview techniques. I was invited to Brunel University in London for an interview and got a place on the course. The car journey in one direction alone took an hour and a half, but I didn't care. A chance is a chance, I thought. I still worked at the hospital and did the course part-time.

'I would have liked having you around back then Mo,' I quipped.

'You weren't paying me back then.' Mo quipped.

'No,' I replied. 'But you are paying now!' I laughed.

'I failed the first year and had to drop out. I carried on working in an assistant role for a while longer before moving to Berlin.

'But I never gave up my dream.' I said.

'I know you didn't. The first week you were in Berlin you did the rounds at local physiotherapy practices asking for an assistant job without even stringing a decent sentence in German together.'

'That was funny, wasn't it?' I replied.

I had to work really hard to learn the German language before I could apply again for physiotherapy. I expected it would take a few years. Eight years later I had another chance. I applied to a school and got in.

Seven months before the course I started pre-learning for up to forty minutes per day while commuting to and from my day job.

'That was full-on!' said Mo.

'I did it because I enjoyed it,' I replied. 'I also got a job as a carer in a nursing home to practice moving and mobilising people in the evening after school had finished.'

'Which you didn't enjoy doing!' said Mo.

'I didn't. But I did the job to learn something new.' I said.

'And it worked.'

'Yeah, it was cool in some respects. I would ask the nurses in charge if they had time to look at my homework,'

'Did they?' asked Mo

'They did. Every staff member I worked with chipped in to help. If I was learning about the heart the head nurse would have me by his side when giving out appropriate heart medications to the residents. He would tell me certain changes I am likely to expect in the elderly and would see typical blood results for this group of people.'

In return, I would show them mobilising techniques I had just learnt at school. We formed a close-knit team. We were actually providing better care for the residents who lived there!

But a lack of skills in the classroom let me down. I didn't pass the first year of the course in Berlin and dropped out, again!

'I was worried you were going to blow a gasket,' said Mo.

'Well, thanks,' I said. 'It was very difficult to deal with failing for the third time. Within a few days, I dropped out of the course.

'However, I wouldn't have done anything differently. I met some great teachers, therapists and patients throughout my entire time in physiotherapy. It is just a shame that success didn't meet me either.'

'So, what happened afterwards?' said Mo.

'I left the carer job because I couldn't use the information I had learnt to good use anymore.'

'That was before your diagnosis, right?' said Mo.

'I was in fact in the diagnosis process when I was studying in Berlin. I was diagnosed with ADHD two months after I dropped out,'

Being tested for a potential mental illness makes even the strongest of us fall to our knees. The stability in my old life was completely gone. I had left my old life and entered into a new one all of a sudden. I was free-falling.

I was embarrassed, I didn't have anyone to talk to about the changes happening to me so I dissected how I felt, what I knew was true to me, in the hope that my self-esteem would improve. I only had myself and wrote for hours to try and see clearly.

I came to the following conclusions.

- I knew I wasn't quick enough to learn lots of information in a short space of time, which was required for the course. I would hit the subject from every angle. Life experience was key. I wanted total immersion and to learn in a drip-feed form.

- I expected to learn from trial and error, adjust slowly to improve any outcome while raising self- esteem.

- I was so embarrassed that I didn't want to speak to my fellow classmates or even see them while going through the ADHD diagnosis.

- I was the first one in the classroom and the last one to leave. (so motivated!)

- During short exams, I would use the allotted time up completely. I would mostly look through the paper if I did have time to spare and check it through like five times. Most people where through small tests in at least half the time and I would always be the last in the room. Would that mean that I didn't know the information? I believe it did.

- I was the oldest person in the class. The one who worked in the field of physiotherapy in two other countries. It almost seemed like a lie!

'What did you realise after your diagnosis?' said Mo.

'Due to my natural state, I was distracted all of the time and couldn't learn properly!'

ADHD is not some kind of superpower. It's one of the most debilitating brain functioning defects there can be. After eight months of tests, my doctor concluded that I didn't have the capacity to concentrate longer than a twenty-minute period.

'That is why being in a classroom for forty-five minutes was never going to work,' said Mo.

'Exactly,' I replied. 'In the hospital I saw patients in twenty-minute slots. That short period fitted me perfectly.'

'You just didn't know!' said Mo amazed.

'I was also told that I couldn't mentally move 3D objects around in my head either to get a correct answer.' I continued.

'But the job of a physiotherapist is to move patients' limbs!'

'True,' I said. 'But it goes deeper than that.'

'If I had a skeleton in front of me, I couldn't name the origin and insertion points of muscles, when asked, even though I had a good grasp of each of their names.'

'Because you couldn't work it out.'

'I couldn't work it out! Interesting, right?' I said to Mo with a smile. 'But I have noticed something that completely goes under our radar.'

'Which is?' said Mo.

'With ADHD we don't pass courses we try really hard for but we sacrifice other areas in our lives for zero *total gain*.'

'What do you mean?' said Mo.

'We have a huge lack of narratives. There is no "do you remember when we used to…?" or "what was that thing that so-and-so said?" because of the overload in our lives. Moreover, we try to pass another course with enthusiasm and effort, but fail again eroding our life away and any further chances of creating more positive narratives for ourselves.'

'Do you still think that you could pass a physiotherapy course if you enrolled for the fourth time?' asked Mo.

I gave the question a few seconds to sink into my brain.

'Yes, I believe that I could still complete a physiotherapy course if I wanted to,' I said to Mo with a smile. 'But I could only do it with you,' I said.

'So, why don't you do it?' asked Mo.

'Because I have found an area that I want to specialise in that loves me more than I love it.'

'That's a bit weird' said Mo.

'I agree. Came out a bit strange, didn't it?' I said.

'Do you mean the ADHD group you formed?'

'And writing a book on the subject,' I added.

'I want to deliver the message, in written form and in person, that adults with ADHD are not broken. They can have a great life and achieve the things that are important to them. That is why I call my group the *ADHD success group*. Being diagnosed with ADHD is the best thing that has ever happened to me.'

'But you are writing a book in English and running an ADHD success group in German. How will that work?' Mo asked.

'I had to change a few things in my head around, thanks mostly to Erin Meyer, but let me take you back to my school days in Berlin. That was a super melting pot for new ideas.'

Principles

- Find an area of work you would love to do as early on in your life as possible.

- If an important goal can be reached on the other side of the world, go for it. The answers to how you can live will come to you. I was fortunate enough that my wife came with me because she believed I could do it.

- Complete work experience or get a part-time job in an area which complements your educational course. You will learn about a topic from a completely different point of view and get to meet some interesting people and be up-to-date with news and skills.

- Life coaches can be brilliant to prepare you for interviews. Find one!

- When applying to an educational establishment. There will always be someone who sees life experience before qualifications. Find them!

- Ask employers if you can work for them 'straight-up' even if you haven't got a qualification. Speaking to the boss, even asking to do anything will put you in the environment you need to be in. Bosses like people who are proactive, I have never been refused a conversation with them because there are really very few people around that make the effort.

- I did pre-learning for every physiotherapy course. Repetition is the key.

- Know your weaknesses. People will tell you these over the years, sometimes quietly. You should also know your strengths. Be prepared to review your strengths and weaknesses after an ADHD diagnosis and with medication. Then concentrate on your strengths!

- Things in life don't work out sometimes. Don't let this upset you. Instead take a pen and paper and write down (when the information is fresh) everything you can to give you a better perspective and to move forward.

- ADHD is not some kind of superpower. It's one of the most debilitating brain functioning defects there can be.

- I didn't have the capacity to concentrate longer than a 20 minute period. I couldn't mentally move 3D objects around in my head. I'm glad I know this now.

- People with undiagnosed ADHD have a huge lack of positive narratives in their lives.

- After the diagnosis stage, and if you have been positive for ADHD go through the 'courteous caving in' stage from Chapter 4.

Chapter Seven – The apprenticeship scheme

Years before my diagnosis, I enrolled onto a three-year apprentice scheme to become an assistant retail manager in the organic food sector in Berlin. The race was on to get a German qualification as my English ones weren't recognised. In a way it was a warm-up before I attempted physiotherapy. If I could pass this sandwich course then I knew better things would come. My second child was born at this time, which was great. Earning some money, getting more involved in the culture but most of all expecting to learn some new and valuable information got me really fired up!

I remember passing teenagers at the entrance of the college on my first day and being mistaken for a new teacher when I couldn't find my classroom. I was, after all, 37 years of age! The students were all so young, they had just finished school. The teachers hit us hard with information from the get-go. They had to prepare the young audience around me for real life. 'During the third lesson on the first day, I was asked to explain the process of photosynthesis. It took me twenty minutes.'

'That must have been fun,' said Mo, sarcastically.

'Well, not really,' I replied.

'I couldn't string a German sentence together properly under pressure so I asked the class for key words that I hadn't even of heard before.'

'And they helped?' asked Mo.

'They were all great,' I replied. 'The stress of keeping poise in a foreign environment is very difficult to do. This went on for months until I got up to speed. I didn't want to fall back on my English so I guess this environment sharpened me up.'

'You couldn't have used your English anyway!' said Mo.

The pressure increased. I could count in German but found it strange saying the numbers backwards. I soon got the hang of it and within two years moulded myself quite well into balancing profit and loss statements.

'I liked being accepted by my class. We never had any problems whatsoever, even though I was a clear thirteen years older than the next oldest member. I appreciated being around teenagers and a handful of adults but all of them were finding themselves in life and their random gestures and immature jokes made me laugh because it was in line with my sense of humour.

'I really liked going to school. Slowly, I would learn about Berlin and Germany from their perspective, hear slang words, understand in great detail how the districts of the city operate and listen in to them speaking amongst themselves as to which apps and mobile phones were the best at that time. I'm sure I learnt more from them then they did from me! I had to write a dash through the number seven when writing financial data. My classmates would laugh at me when I would write the number seven the English way and think it was the number one.

'The teacher would get annoyed when I used a dot instead of a comma. If the comma was used incorrectly, I would be asking for millions and not thousands of euros when submitting a business plan to a bank. I didn't quite believe them, so in typical Simon style I tested this theory out when working at the shop. I found that if I manually inputted an item for ten euros into a German till and wrote 10.00 the computer didn't recognise the "dot" and would take this value as 1000 euros! But it wasn't just the numbers that had to be correct.

'I would construct a spoken sentence with the verb at the end instead of at the front of a sentence. I would have to persuade a class full of people that the new business venture of mine is worthwhile. I couldn't state the fact of the matter first but instead had to build up a theoretical concept for the class to analyse.

'I learnt very early on from Erin Meyer that my "…habitual pattern of reasoning is heavily influenced by the kind of thinking emphasized in your culture's educational structure."' (2014: 93/94)

'Was that difficult for you?' asked Mo.

'It was just plain different, that's all,' I said. 'Remember, I would be submerged in this environment and I don't mean just at school, I mean generally.'

'So that helped?' asked Mo.

'You cannot beat living in a country to pick up the culture, but I had to look at how I was communicating in the first place.' I answered 'There is something called the Applications-first theory. I was bought up using this in the UK.'

'Which is what?' asked Mo.

'Erin states that "individuals are trained to begin with a fact, statement or opinion and later add concepts to back up or explain the conclusion as necessary".' (2014: 96)

'I then changed to a principles-first theory, which means "Individuals have been trained to first develop the theory or complex concept before presenting a fact, statement or opinion".' (2014: 96)

'So, the other way around!' said Mo.

'I guess so,' I said. 'After all, the German language is spoken and written the other way round to English.'

'Erin suggests, "Presenting to French, Spaniards, or Germans? Spend more time setting the parameters and explaining the background before jumping to your conclusion".' (2014: 101)

'So you used that in a school environment?' asked Mo.

'Yes. I got that under my belt after a while.'

'So, you use this approach now for the ADHD success group?'

'Exactly,' I said. 'But it was trickier to work in the shop environment.'

'You didn't talk that much when you worked at the till,' said Mo.

'I don't mean that,' I said. 'There is something called task-based trust, which has to do with business related activities. If you do work consistently, you are reliable.'

'I see,' said Mo.

'Yes,' I replied, as if looking into my own self to promote the point.

I honestly took Erin Meyers book on the train with me to work every single day. I would read through a few chapters over again so I wouldn't step out of line.

'In the UK, Germany and in Australia where I have lived and worked, task-based trust was everything! With undiagnosed ADHD task-based trust is close to impossible. I needed to be reliable at work and I wasn't.'

'That's why people with ADHD have a scattered CV,' said Mo.

'Exactly, because employers see people like me as a 'live wire!'

'But you were bought up in England.' said Mo.

'I know, but that doesn't mean I knew how to integrate!' I replied

'Aha, so you are suggesting that people with ADHD cannot integrate into their own culture,' asked Mo.

'In a way, yes!' I replied.

'So how did you get around this with undiagnosed ADHD?'

'I just needed to chop cultures down the middle in certain situations to get the results I wanted!'

'Which is pretty difficult because of the lack of your executive functions,'

'True, Mo, but don't forget, I didn't know that before! I only knew about the problems I was having with ADHD after a I listened to Dr Russell Barkley's audio book called *Taking Charge of Adult ADHD*.'

'But that was ages ago.'

'Yes, it was five years before my diagnosis.'

'You waited that long?' said Mo.

'Yeah. I was second guessing myself for a long time. I felt I needed all of the facts on this subject before going for a diagnosis.'

'And you took notes?' asked Mo.

'On what?' I asked.

'On areas that could be useful to you in the future.' said Mo.

'Oh, I have always been doing that,' I replied.

'So, keeping up-to-date?' said Mo.

'Yes, I believe so.'

'But you looked to Erin for more advice,' said Mo.

'I couldn't have worked out so many areas of life without her research,' I said. 'I felt I had to try and fit in aggressively in Berlin during the early days because I saw that as the norm! I would love to meet Erin and tell her what new discovery I made.'

'Which is?' said Mo.

'Since I have taken medication, I have an awareness now which brings me more into line with the German culture,' I said.

'How come?' asked Mo.

'I went through each section of her book and plotted my own assessment of how I have changed since medication.'

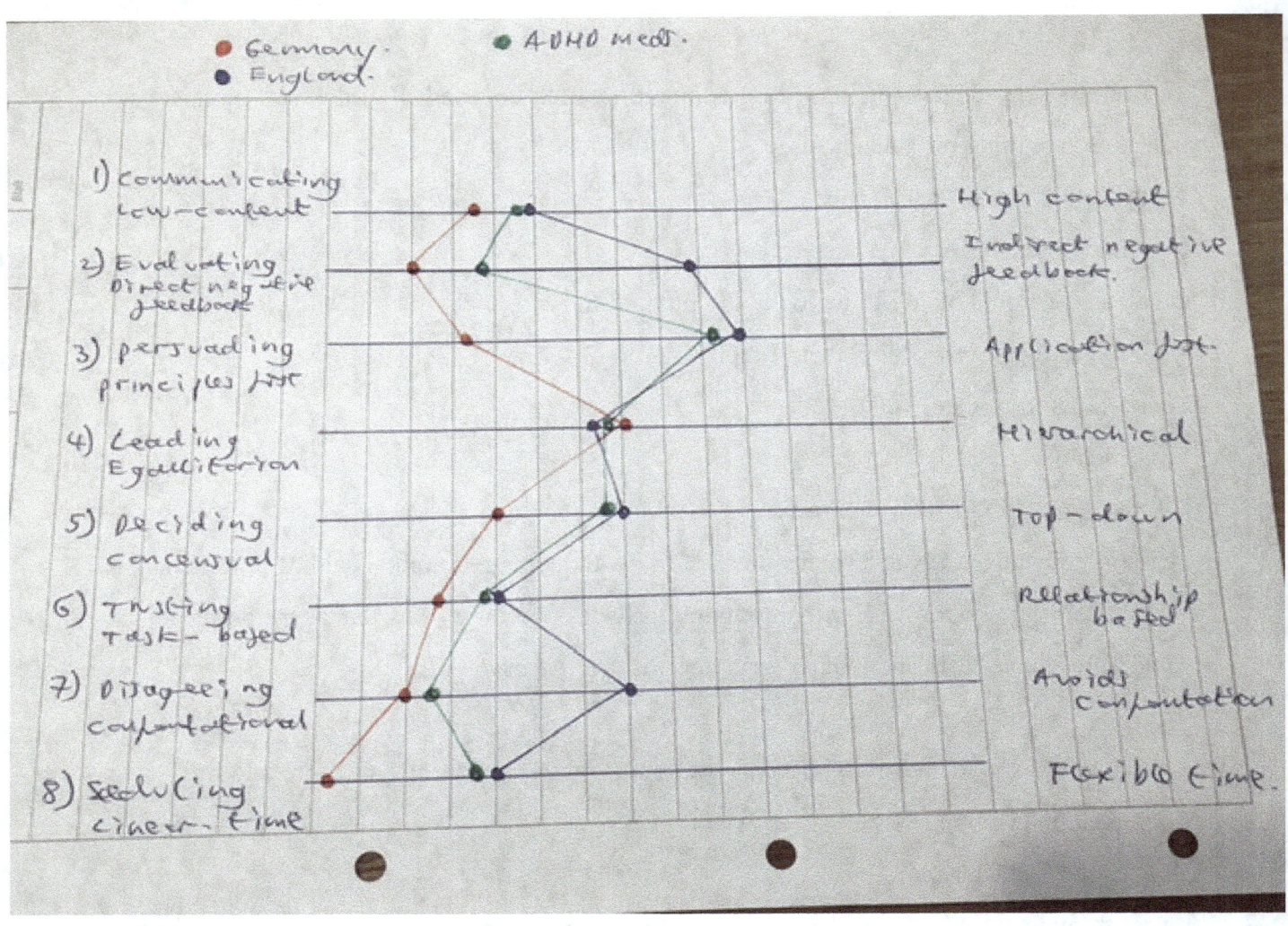

'For example, I was doing much better in the area of "disagreeing", which brings me more in line with this country. I just have to remember that when I go back to the UK to see family that I don't knock them off of their stool with the way I converse now!'

'So, coming over too confrontational?' asked Mo.

'Yes,' I replied. 'Moreover, the school environment moulded me slowly into the workings of this country in quite a big way. At the shop, I soaked up things like a sponge and somehow fitted in. I narrowly passed the course after the three-year period being the third person with an English nationality in the school's history to do so.'

'So you did complete something!' said Mo.

'I did, but I only just scraped through,' I said.

As an older person, I see that the average person in society has experienced school, passed exams and is busy working for a company or for themselves. For many, that is the last time they see a learning environment. They open themselves up for grander things in life such as finding a partner, having kids, travelling or moving up the career ladder. They can build their lives purely from the qualification they have achieved. They have got to first base.

But, ADHD is very disabling. I never wanted to go back to a school environment and constantly feel like I was starting from the bottom again. I have done this so many times.

Now that I take medication, I can do the things that everyone else (healthy people) did twenty years ago. I am only realising what works now with my switched-on brain. I have a twenty-year lag.

I got my head around this concept and accepted it.

'Adults with ADHD have a terrible time learning so I titled up a new area of interest. I called this area "Understanding the basics of a class-based learning environment and learning with ADHD".'

'That sounds exciting,' said Mo.

'It's probably what really started my meet-up group off properly in the first place,' I said.

Principles

- Complete a course that gives you a higher chance of employment. This will prime you for what you really want to do later.

- Ask younger people than yourself for assistance in a class environment when you need it. Count on them. Learn from them!

- The way you explain something to an audience may not be the right way. Adapt.

- Applications-first theory: "Individuals are trained to begin with a fact, statement or opinion and later add concepts to back up or explain the conclusion as necessary.

- Principles-first theory: "Individuals have been trained to first develop the theory or complex concept before presenting a fact, statement or opinion." See Meyer (2014) for more information.

- Task-based trust is how people see reliability of someone in the workplace in specific countries.

- With undiagnosed ADHD, task-based trust is impossible. That's why people with ADHD have a scattered CV.

- I believe it is difficult for a person with ADHD to assimilate into their own country.

- Medication can help a person adjust to society.

- Having ADHD may result in you starting from the bottom of the career ladder. You too could have a twenty-year lag. If you are diagnosed, at least you know this now!

Chapter Eight – Understanding the basics of a class-based learning environment and learning with ADHD

If you have ADHD and need to go back to school to get a qualification, first and foremost you have to want to be at the school. The qualification you are working for will come easier to those who want to put the work in. Second, try and sit at the front of the class. You will be able to see the white board and hear the teacher. Keep quiet and observe your new class-mates. If you have made yourself comfortable in your new surroundings on the first day attempt to ground yourself.

I know there are some of you that don't use ADHD medication and I applaud you for that. Medication isn't right for everyone. However, just bear in mind that whispering happens in classrooms, no matter what age the group is. It will be on the same loudness level of everything else and you don't want to ask the teacher to repeat what they have just said.

'How should people steer themselves with a new personality? That can be hard to do, I imagine.' asked Mo.

'Well,' I replied. 'You may find you are quieter than before, which has advantages in the classroom; after all, you don't want to come over as a know-it-all and/or take up the lion's share of the teacher's time.

'But be aware that during break times you could come over to others as being uninterested, rude or just in your own world. It is probably good to take your eyes away from a mobile phone device during break time and perhaps play a game of pool or something similar, get some fresh air or speak with others.'

If you are concerned about fitting in with your class members just remember this quote from Jack Canfield:

"Most of the time, nobody is thinking about you at all! They are too busy worrying about their own lives, and if they are thinking about you at all, they are wondering what you are thinking about them. People think about themselves, not you." (2005: 69)

'Do you think people with ADHD can start to really enjoy studying a subject now?' asked Mo.

'Yes, I do, but if you are the type of person who is motivated to learn then the added new perception you have now can bring you good dividends,' I replied. 'Making decisions should be a lot easier for people who are now treated and have ADHD.'

'What do you mean?' said Mo, 'Deciding what you want to eat for lunch?' he said with a laugh.

'Yes, you can do that anyway,' I grinned back at myself, 'but I mean deciding intentionally to stay quiet in a very particular situation.'

'Can't wait to hear this,' said Mo.

'During a discussion of a topic which involves the whole class and can take a few hours to complete – just be quiet.'

'But you couldn't!' said Mo.

'I had a horrible habit, before I was diagnosed (over 42 years!), of asking a question when the teacher was in full swing.'

'What's wrong with that?' enquired Mo.

'Nothing really, but my question was relevant ten minutes before!'

'That's weird,' said Mo. 'I bet you got ridiculed for that.'

'I did. I felt I was like being pulled over the coals.'

Dr Russell Barkley says "You're no child, but these lags make you less effective than other adults and may make your peers treat you as if you were a child." (2010: 71)

'But I was asking a question to gain more understanding.'

'Instead of listening completely to what the teacher was saying,' Mo said, chipping in.

'Yes, but when we discussed *real world* topics in relation to the material we were studying, I couldn't help myself because I spent loads of time in the real working world. Do you see my dilemma?

'I got bad looks in Australia, England and Germany for just jumping in! It wasn't a language problem. I had been doing this my whole life and thought it was normal, until I saw it wasn't.'

'Was it impulse driven?' asked Mo.

'Yes, I was trying to tie in information I was learning in the present with past life experience. I actually now see that when others asked a question it was relevant for that exact time period of the discussion, so it fit. Class members were mostly quiet otherwise.'

'But you were showing initiative,' interrupted Mo.

'…Yes, and falling on my face in the meantime.'

A learning environment is also naturally competitive. Classmates would give quicker answers than I could and people would finish or rephrase my sentences when I asked a question. The teachers couldn't understand what I *meant* to say. Then another person in the class chips in saying 'I think Simon was meant to say is this,' and formulates it much better and an answer is given. But this process was excruciatingly painful, it wastes time and lowers your value as a class member.

'But that was just in Germany, right?' asked Mo.

'I think it always happened,' I replied.

In the classroom I would only be measured as a therapist if I gave correct answers.

There was no time to have half-baked ideas and to smooth out the answer from the teacher to get a better understanding. That would have meant one-to-one coaching and a class environment isn't like this. I just thought being in different areas of physiotherapy was the best start I could have. But it left me too open. I wasn't ready to be so confined into a subject area that when I said just one word out of place it would have been wrong. This, I get in a class environment but the world out there doesn't work like that. Every case you see isn't a 'text book' answer. It cannot be!

The experience in the hospital environment was not relevant. I wasn't trying to fake myself to success. Moreover, I had all of my first-year physiotherapy notes from Brunel University – I didn't want to pre-learn every single piece of information required to complete a physiotherapy course before I started another one. People in the learning environment then started to distrust me. I was keen and, in some cases, 'overly keen'. It seems to many that I am just 'full of myself' when in fact I'm not. It's the mix between my twenty-something outlook and the need to improve things that don't work. I don't fall into the middle of the society that everyone understands, but honestly, the middle of society is not where the magic happens. It is always on the edges.

The point is, I knew that a whole lifetime of high motivation didn't even scratch the surface of what I wanted to accomplish. Just the feeling of life being stacked up on me, that everything in my environment was always at the loudest setting could drop a normal person into a huge hole that screaming cannot bring you out of.

This is why undiagnosed ADHD kills us dead in our tracks if we let it. This is why this book has been written. People in our society need to know that ADHD can carry on into adulthood.

'It just doesn't magically stop when a seventeen-year-old kid with ADHD has his eighteenth birthday!'

'Although, that would be nice, wouldn't it?' said Mo.

'But I noticed a very interesting comment from students being made every time examinations were approaching.'

'Which was?' said Mo.

'"I hope I don't black out," someone would say followed by a typical answer from a class-mate such as, "You know the stuff, you will okay."

'That scenario stuck with me one day. I don't think I ever could ever have a *black out* I con-cluded. I was, up until now, always living in the present. I had no recall. I couldn't grasp the past information I had learnt because of lack of certain executive functions.'

'Now fast forward to having being diagnosed and taking medication. Imagine you have now been given a map so you can respond fast and with accuracy at the right time. I admit that is seems unreal at first but you soon catch on.'

'There is nothing better than saying goodbye to Mr or Mrs Scatterbrain who is ten minutes behind,' said Mo.

'That's a good one,' I said.

'But it could well be that we can have a blackout now. I just haven't tested it out.'

You should have a better concept with organising paperwork but approach someone you know for tips and tricks if they can do it well. You should be able to recognise these people simply by scanning the neater folders left on desks during your break time. Although you can finish jobs off now, slip ups will happen, so learn to recognise them.

You should find that consistent time spent in the classroom combined with a balanced concept of good brain function, recognising distractions and actively ignoring them will in-crease your self-esteem in the short and long term. You are less likely to be treated differ-ently.

I took 100% responsibility for my ADHD. Then I seriously had to work on self-care. There was the aspect of stigmatism that I was feeling from others. I started writing tips and tricks to make ADHD manageable. This is where the real intensity of note taking turned into journal-ing. I decided to paint my life in colour. I slowly knew myself, because I was the person I would spend most of my time with!

'You may find that the person in the classroom who helps you organise your papers could be a good study partner too. These are the people that light up a room when they enter it, they almost always have a smile on their face, have time for others even though they are busy, have a great personality and work hard at what they do.'

'Which leads us on to your meet-up group,' said Mo.

I started an ADHD success group to drive people with the condition forward, while creating a solid base of support. But before I even started the first meeting, I knew I wasn't the best person in a social situation. I had to look at this area before I could make my group a huge success.

Principles

- You must want to learn when you enrol onto a course. The qualification you are working for will come easier. Also, sit at the front of the class.

- Constant whispering in a class environment is an indicator that people are not interested in learning or find the course too easy. However, whispering is very loud and disruptive to our ears with undiagnosed ADHD. With medication I find it tolerable.

- If you don't understand something, ask your classmates. They make be able to help you! (even those that have been whispering!). A study partner will be beneficial.

- Have you asked a question that was relevant ten minutes prior? Can you get to the bottom of why you do this? Try by yourself or seek professional advice.

- Does the following quote ring true with you "You're no child, but these lags make you less effective than other adults and may make your peers treat you as if you were a child." (Barkley, 2010: 71). Seek help if you know this is true.

- A class-based environment is competitive – don't forget that.

- I knew that since I was twenty years old, a high motivation didn't even scratch the surface of what I wanted to accomplish. How many years do you want to wait? I waited twenty-two years!!! This is why undiagnosed ADHD kills us dead in our tracks if we let it.

- I believe it isn't possible to have a 'black out' during exams with undiagnosed ADHD. I had no recall due to certain executive functions. On medication it could now be possible. Reduce your stress levels. Work with supporting classmates on the subject of interest and when an exam comes up be happy that your working memory is now up to speed.

- Glance at the folders on the desks. Who is neat? Who is organised? Ask them how they file correctly. You can do this now! Just ask.

- Take 100% responsibility for your ADHD.

- Write your own notes about your ADHD. This will make you feel better. I would love to read them too!

- Decide to paint your life in colour. You will slowly know yourself, because you are the person you spend most of your time with!

Chapter Nine – Socialising

A lady in her thirties opened up a conversation with me one day about how difficult it is in Berlin to make friendships. She was German, had two toddlers at kindergarten and would regularly sit at playgrounds in the afternoon when nursery had finished. Week after week, she would see the same mums and some dads in the vicinity watching their kids play. It took a couple of years before anyone really had a conversation with her. She suggested that people need to let a good amount of time pass so that friendships can be developed slowly and properly. 'I had to be patient because people do keep to themselves,' she said.

'That makes sense,' I told her.

But I couldn't fathom out why friendships take so long to even start! So after a shift at work one day, I looked into this a little more. I knew from my own heritage that there is a blur of mixing business and pleasure. Even the moral of the gingerbread boy story is *we should not trust anyone without consideration.* Remember, he got eaten in the end and we don't want the same happening to ourselves! But judging situations completely wrong in the past puts people with ADHD at a real disadvantage. Until now.

If you are anything like me, you have a great deal of impatience. We can now use it to our advantage. Our impatience can deter us naturally from people that aren't good for us. As more and more people live abroad, like me, it is essential to give these particular people in that country, who don't see us as equal, a wide berth (until I have worked how to go about it in a better way and write about it in my next book!).

One day, I asked a friend of mine who is a university lecturer how to socialise. I admitted I had no filter whatsoever with the information coming out of my mouth. I presumed that being completely open was normal until I said something that was totally inappropriate for his ears.

'We only knew each other for four weeks.'

'That is too short a period of time,' said Mo.

'Yes, it definitely is,' I agreed.

'He was in reality, someone you just got to know, instead of a friend,' said Mo.

'I asked him what he doesn't do in a social context. He replied, "we don't need to tell everyone everything about our lives". So, I went home, grabbed some colouring pens from my kids and came up with this picture-gram of how I perceived myself to be!

Undiagnosed ADHD person

Grey indicates the stuff you know about me. Top layer is what you
know about me and the bottom is what you don´t.

Verdict: Too transparent with information. All information is given out.
knowing at least 90% of someone is too much for anyone. There is no
gauge as to what is too much information and where privacy starts.

Atypical person (no ADHD)

Blue indicates the stuff you know about a person or what
they tell you about themselves.
Green indicates the information you don't know about a person. Their protection of their own information.
Their security of themselves.

Verdict: Shows individualism and is healthy. People
shouldn't know more than 50% about you.

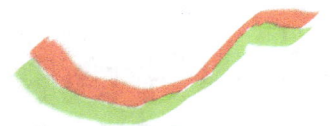

ADHD Person on medication (1st year).

Red indicates the information you know about me and also the things I tell you about myself. It is in red because I am at the cautious stage. I am building up my mental muscles, my life shield and my identity.
Green indicates the information you don't know about me and that of information that is now not forthcoming. Red 70%
Green 30%

Verdict: I am forming my new self

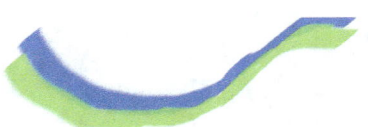

ADHD person on medication (1 year or longer)

Blue indicates the information you know about me and also the things I tell you about myself. It is now blue because I have solidified these areas and I am comfortable.
Green indicates the information you don't know about me and that of information that is not forthcoming.

Verdict: I have a healthy 50/50 transparency while also protecting my privacy.

'I also hadn't heard of *social interaction* classes that people can attend so I had to work things out for myself when more than one person in an environment is present.'

'You had to get to a social gathering on time, first,' said Mo.

'True, I was late quite often,' I said. 'When I chose to be punctual for the coming week, that was where my effort went. I believed that if I could choose a small area and hone in on it then one day all the areas will fall into place. But I think it turned into a habit, regardless of the ADHD. The habit stuck. Then after a while you build up such an array of good habits in singular areas. Then when medicated and the brain works properly it seems you can effortlessly do things well in the mind of others.'

'Because you combine all of the areas together? Is that what you mean?' asked Mo.

'Yeah, but I always wondered if people with neurotypical brains had no need to develop each individual area because they could orchestrate these areas "normally".'

'I guess you will never know.'

'Perhaps,' I replied.

'Your wife's suggestion of using a stop watch with a capped time limit was a good idea,' said Mo.

'Yeah, the six-minute talk-and-then-shut-up'rule,' I laughed.

'Well, it worked, didn't it?'

'Yes,' I replied.

'One day, you were talking to a lady at a social event and her eyes were slowly closing,' Mo quipped.

'What is that supposed to mean?' I asked.

'You were boring the hell out of her!'

'No I wasn't,' I replied in haste.

'But you didn't join in with the group of people at the table, did you?' said Mo. 'You single people out.'

'That's a bit harsh,' I finished.

I realised I couldn't follow a conversation in a group of more than three people if I was the fourth. Therefore, I would have never fitted into a group, even if I wanted to. This happened in any situation, be it conversing with friends, family or at work. Following dialogue was difficult because of environmental noise. Ever since I was child, my grandmother said over and over again *treat people how you to want to be treated*. I have done that. I have a few close friends, but I overdo it every single time when trying to make new ones.

I become far too close or far too distant. I am upfront and honest. Erin Meyer wrote,

"Kurt Lewin was one of the first social scientists to explain individual personality as being partially formed by the cultural system in which a person is raised. Authors Fons Trompenaars and Charles Hampden-Turner later expanded on Lewin's model to explain how different cultures have different layers of information that they divulge publicly or reserve for private relationships. These models are referred to as the peach and coconut models of personal interaction." (2014: 175)

'I had read about the peach and coconut model years ago,' I told Mo.

Erin Meyer describes the peach culture as people who

"…smile frequently at strangers, move quickly to first name usage, share information about themselves and ask personal questions of those they hardly know. But after a little friendly interaction with a peach person, you may suddenly get to the hard shell of the pit where the peach protects his real self. In these cultures, friendliness does not equal friendship." (2014: 175–176)

On the other hand, when I moved to Berlin, Germany, the culture is different.

Erin suggests, "In coconut cultures…people are more closed (like the tough shell of a coconut) with those they don't have friendships with…" continuing, "It takes a while to get through the initial hard shell, but as you do, people will become gradually warmer and friendlier." (Meyer, 2014: 177)

But Berlin has an antagonistic element too. "In more confrontational cultures, it seems quite natural to attack someone's opinion without attacking that person." (2014: 200)

'And were you working out all of these complexities at once?' asked Mo.

'Yes,' I replied, 'I found it really quite fun.'

The problem with undiagnosed ADHD is that it's very difficult to recall past experiences so we launch into the same environment again and again getting the same results.

'Perhaps you can help me, Mo?' I asked.

'Yes, of course,' he said 'What's up?'

'I know I am very good at destroying any kind of social relationship, but how would you distinguish when something isn't important compared to something that is, and behaving accordingly?'

'Well,' said Mo. 'I guess most people have to filter the information they experience. I can only assume that your brain, before the diagnosis was running at *light-speed*. You had no way to slow it down and would be mentally falling over yourself.

'When someone speaks to you individually this gives your brain a rest,' said Mo. 'You like that rest so you then want more of it. Then you get emotionally involved. You can't see the *normal connection*. You can use this emotion to an advantage to learn things, get geared up and to do the best job but it is rubbish for social interactions. After a while the emotion is then pre-set. You then cannot tell anymore that it this your driving force. You need to go into situations with an emotional free element and that will take some time to get used to.'

'I'm not in a rush to work this out,' I replied. 'Mo, I am writing this book to feel a part of society. People have always said to me 'You talk too much, you are bullshitting, you explain too much of yourself, you have these great ideas but never get anywhere! You are still in school or better yet, you didn't pass *anything!*'

Before medication I was always in survival mode. I would go into a new friendship and would soon end up arguing with them over something unimportant and not want to talk with them. I would then delete their phone number and all of their messages because, don't forget, I only lived in the present. I didn't have the option to see the good times we had or the moments we could enjoy in a week, month or year's time from now.

A certain amount of time would go by. If they write back, then I know we are on good terms and is my chance then to secure the relationship. I have really good friends that know I have ADHD but it is due to their flexibility that they stick with me.

'On the plus side, if they are having a hard time, I can give them totally abstract ideas that they have never thought of to help them through. It is like I am their *mad scientist* friend!'

'But you are really impatient, Simon,' said Mo.

'Only in certain situations,' I said. 'I have never understood in a social or work environment if a question that has been asked needs an immediate response. I always wanted to give an answer right away, just like any teacher wanted from me in the classroom.'

'You treated *like* with *like*.' said Mo.

'Exactly.' I replied. 'I felt that in Germany people are over accurate with everything.'

'I know exactly why you think that way,' said Mo.

'Pray, tell,' I said.

'You feel you need to fit in. You feel you need to make up for lost time.'

'So I should slow down?' I asked Mo.

'You choose yourself first and foremost and not to go to every social setting that is presented, even if people really want you to go.'

'I'll do that,' I said to Mo.

'I am finally making connections and am living so much more than before. I think this is the time that I can have real and meaningful personal relationships for the first time in my life. To know just from eye contact I will bring across trust, attention and a willingness to be interested in what the person is saying. To see people's eye colour for the first time, to know that a certain person has blue eyes which make small alterations in colours due to the shining sun.'

'That is the good part of experiencing life,' said MO.

'Can you remember the quote from the book, the *Chronicles from the Future*, Mo?'

'"I cast these bad thoughts out and wandered into the crowd feeling as if I fit in again, like I belonged in their world. At least that's what my physical appearance said – without betraying anything of what was happening inside me – and that made me swell with pride! I did, however, wonder whether the joy and happiness I felt was ultimately non-existent, whether it was nothing more than mere enthusiasm.",' I said. (Dienach, 2018: 145)

But you are working on this area,' said Mo.

'I am,' I said 'and I will get there.'

'Again, you just have to slow down a touch, and keep conversations like that very basic,' said Mo. You should also not expect an answer immediately from a text message you sent to someone, an email, a post on a social networking site.'

'Ok, I get it Mo,' I said.

'But now in a group environment I have difficulty seeing all of the people around me when I use medication,' I said to Mo.

'How come?' said Mo.

'Well, I noticed I had a problem with my eyesight at the far peripheral range.'

'What do you mean by far peripheral range?' asked Mo.

'Years ago, when I worked as a physiotherapy assistant, we had glasses in the department to give us an understanding of patients with eyesight issues. These glasses decreased a person's vision in some way or another.'

'Get it.'

'Far peripheral vision is the area of sight between 60 degrees and 100 to 110 degrees, so basically the area to your furthest right or left when you keep your head straight.'

'So you can't see people in this range?' said Mo.

'I am not blind in this range, but I don't see people or objects. If people say something and I'm positioned in this range it surprises me.'

'Is it any easier after a year on medication?' asked Mo.

'No, not really,' I said.

'I guess it what people called hyper-focus,' said Mo 'You have to do the best you can.'

'I then realised I should understand relationships before I start the success group. Socialising and relationships go hand in hand.'

'But why relationships?' said Mo.

'You only have to socialise with the people from your group, you don't want to go out with them!' he laughed.

'Very funny Mo,' I said.

'I think, if I can round off my knowledge in the area of relationships, I can then hold seminars later on in this area for people with ADHD who need answers as much as I did.'

'Good point,' said Mo.

'I want to act decisively to whatever topic we discuss when I am in a leadership position. A leader is a leader for a reason.' I finished.

Jack Canfield wrote, "Once you begin to respond quickly and decisively to signals and events as they occur, life becomes much easier". (2005: 23)

We live in a world where people are spending more time on media and dating apps.

I have seen first-hand that many people with ADHD are going it alone. But what if I have found a few answers that can help in the area of relationships? This is what I found out through books and my own study of the area.

Principles

- It takes a couple of years to get to know anyone. Why? We should not trust anyone without consideration (from the Gingerbread boy).
- Our impatience can deter us naturally from people that aren't good for us.
- Don't be afraid to ask people how you come over in situations. Then reflect on it.
- We don't need to tell everyone everything about our lives.
- Keep to a healthy 50/50 of the information you give out about yourself and of that that is secret. It is not too much or not too little. I need medication to keep to this 50/50 level.

- Use a stop watch or timer when in conversation with others so you don't take over a whole conversation (the six-minute talk-and-then-shut-up- rule).
- I couldn't follow a conversation in a group of more than three people if I was the fourth. This happened in any situation because of environmental noise.
- Understand social rules of those people in your life whose heritage is different to yours. It is very difficult with undiagnosed ADHD. With diagnosed ADHD you can remember what to do and not what to do!
- I couldn't filter information in social relationships. My brain was running at light-speed, I couldn't slow it down and I would be mentally falling over myself. Medication changed all of that. I was bought into line.
- Before medication I was always in survival mode.
- You choose yourself first and foremost and not to go to every social setting that is presented, even if people really want you to go.
- With ADHD, or think you do have it, slow down a touch, and keep conversations very basic.
- When you talk or text or even email people allow much more time for the person to respond to you.
- Far peripheral vision is the area of sight between 60 degrees and 100–110 degrees. Realise that this has to do with the hyper-focus of your eyes. You may be surprised when people come into this range and you do not initially see them. Just so you know!

Chapter Ten – Relationships

Everyone has good and bad relationships with people. That is normal. But I wanted to feel better, much better.

I grabbed all of my diaries out of the cupboard (again), a pen and paper and drew boxes for marriage, family, and working relationships. I made a list of people who made me feel bad but later added a box indicating my own connection to ADHD.

'I bet the marriage box was huge!' laughed Mo.

'Just be quiet.' I said. 'When I was done, I stood before my wife and swore there and then that I will never see the people who make me feel bad again.

'I then took off my wedding ring!'

'You did *what*?' said Mo.

'I needed to get to know myself. I couldn't envisage wearing it and supporting my family if this area wasn't looked at.'

'That's a bit drastic,' said Mo.

'Tackling ADHD is always a personal battle.' I replied.

'But you are married!' said Mo outraged.

'Well, you definitely felt the overwhelming feeling of guilt I had for the last couple of months, right!'

'I did, and I didn't like it,' said Mo.

'How often would I say to my wife, "It's probably best if you leave me and go and find someone else without ADHD to make your life so much easier. You haven't deserved this."? Mo was quiet.

'But I wanted to stay married. That was the point. I was just really vulnerable. I was reaching out for help! We needed to restart the relationship again.'

'Which isn't easy,' said Mo.

'It is very hard, Mo. I wanted to know the finer points of the human condition to have a new balanced approach in my marriage and to improve family life together.'

I read the book *Attached* by Dr Amir levine and Rachael S.F Heller M.A to understand the three different attachment styles within romantic relationships. These are secure, anxious and avoidant.

> "…*secure* people feel comfortable with intimacy and are usually warm and loving; *anxious* people crave intimacy, are often preoccupied with their relationships, and tend to

worry about their partner´s ability to love them back; *avoidant* people equate   intimacy with a loss of independence and constantly try to minimize closeness." (Levine & Heller, 2010: 8)

'I have to stress that the *Attached* book is aimed at the general public and is not at all connected or in association with ADHD. I just thought it would be worth looking at.'

'Point made.' said Mo.

'I knew the dynamics of my attachment style had shifted, but how? I completed the questionnaire in the book to see where I landed on the secure, anxious and avoidant scale and wasn't surprised. My ratings were (in order and out of 100%) 50, 75 and 15, respectively. I was very confident that the more I understand ADHD and take my medication my secure rating will slowly go up, the anxiousness and avoidance will go down and that's a good thing!'

'But what happens when ADHD partners increase their stability rating?' asked Mo.

'This is when things get interesting,' I reply. 'They are then more valuable to the relationship.'

'That's great,' said Mo.

'The partner will see improvements, making the relationship as a whole so much more pleasant. I truly believe a new found love with the person you are with can come out of such a situation.'

'You will see this first, in your relationship,' said Mo.

'I'm looking forward to that,' I reply.

'But you have different angles to work with.' said Mo.

'True. Many pages of my diaries were filled with uncomfortable experiences from living in a different country with a new culture and language, which played in with interactions with my wife,'

'Which forced you down a certain route,' said Mo.

'Yes. There is a great quote in the *Attached* book that reads "Another option in a harsh environment is to act in the opposite manner and be intensely persistent and hypervigilant about staying close to your attachment figure (hence the anxious attachment style)." (Levine & Heller, 2010: 13).

'I believe I became dependent on my wife to a huge extent because for many years I couldn't speak the language at a native level. I also became even more dependant as my outside environment (with ADHD) traps me within myself!'

'Oh, my goodness,' said Mo.

'Fast forward a few years and a few German lessons later, and I got a clearer perspective.'

"In a more peaceful setting, the intimate bonds formed by investing greatly in a particular individual would yield greater benefits for both the individual and his or her offspring (hence, the secure attachment style)." (Levine & Heller, 2010: 13)

'So this is what you are working on?' said Mo.

'Yes, I am, and it will take some time,' I replied.

'Fair enough,' said Mo.

'While attending an ADHD self-help clinic at the time I was going through my own diagnosis I listened to stories of others. ADHD in a partnership is difficult but acceptance of ADHD from either party in the partnership plays an important role as well.'

'Where you worried that you felt your wife was doing *everything* for you?' asked Mo.

'No, but quite honestly I would let some things slip.'

'I knew, by default I had a good skill mix. I actually asked my wife what qualities I have without medication because I couldn't see them.'

'Which is a good idea,' said Mo.

'Yeah, when I was medicated, I asked again.'

'That's pretty good to ask again!' said Mo.

'Well, don't forget, I live in a country with a different mentality and different expectations. I guess I got the idea from Jack Canfield, who wrote,

> "Don't be afraid to ask. Most people are afraid to ask for feedback about how they are doing because they are afraid of what they are going to hear. There is nothing to be

afraid of. The truth is the truth. You are better off knowing the truth than not knowing   it."' (2005: 24)

'Did you consider that ADHD could end your marriage?' asked Mo.

'No, Marriages break down because of ADHD, but marriages break down for lots of reasons. Moreover, it doesn't mean that every person with newly diagnosed ADHD will remain single or alone – far from it!'

'Can you imagine if two people with ADHD met?' said Mo.

'Wouldn't it be great if the two of them could increase their secure zone together?' I replied, smiling.

'That sounds utterly romantic,' said Mo.

'So, what about family relationships?' said Mo.

'Of course, we cannot choose our family, we should always be polite to everyone, even those that make us feel bad, but spend as little time with them as possible. I don't need to give my power away to anyone anymore. I can help protect myself, don't mull over worries, and will speak directly to someone if I feel there is bad air between us. I make this quick and concise and decide not to ruin my day over it.'

If all else fails I would remove myself from the situations I am not happy to be in.

'That's a bold move.' said Mo.

'I guess people with ADHD are used to being bold. Earlier I said that it is very difficult to assimilate to any given culture, even one we have been born and grow up in.' I just talk about simple things now, even with the family!'

'But I was seeing before my very eyes certain grievances disappear into thin air.'

'What do you mean by grievances?' said Mo.

'The very area that Russell A. Barkley brings up in his book, such as insufficient planning, impatience, impulsiveness in relationships, interrupting conversations, insufficient coping skills and distractions. Once I knew these areas were significantly reduced or had disappeared, then family issues are much easier to deal with.'

'What you are writing about is definitely not standard book material.' said Mo.

'But if they work for me, it could also work for others too, right?' I said with a smile.

I now know it takes an extraordinary amount of time for us with ADHD to wait for anything, especially the time to build up relationships. And I don't care how others do it either. A messy way to get good results is okay.

One night, my wife asked me about working relationships.

'We spoke for a while about the difficulty of maintaining good working relationships with ADHD.'

'And what did you talk about?' asked Mo.

'ADHD is not just difficult for the person who has it, but can be a battle for those you work with too. I would turn up in the same physical body to my place of work but my personality was completely different.'

'That is weird,' said Mo.

'But it happens overnight,' I said. 'The thing is, the person with ADHD is so busy with their new world they need time to level out.'

'And that is not permitted, I don't understand.' said Mo.

Like I said earlier, 'I can decide what to react to now, and people aren't used to that. There is no trial run in the working world!'

'The people who know you are shocked and need to accept someone different. It scares them.'

'So everything collapses,' suggested Mo.

'Yes, but although it is very uncomfortable in the moment, I knew I could build bigger and better.'

'Because your inner secure rating has increased?' asked Mo

'Exactly. You need to be strong on the inside to move forward in life!'

'Obviously people out there cannot possibly like every staff member they work with. So, I invented the full stop phase.'

'What is that?' asked Mo.

'It is like "courteous caving in" but over a longer period of time. I had to see situations and people as they were over a period of a few weeks. I just decided to use the correct temperament around them.'

'To give you more clarity,' said Mo.

'Yes.' I replied. 'I was being tested constantly. I was performing much better at work. I was completing tasks to the end.'

'I see a "but" coming,' said Mo.

'It gives people the *illusion* that my life is miraculously in order.'

'But it is!' said Mo.

'Yes, but only when the medication is *working*,' I replied. 'It would be a disaster if I turned up to work without medication.'

'Just down to the three reasons for having ADHD in the first place proves that you are dependent on the medication,' said Mo.

'Yes. It is essential to my life. I have heard from others that when they have visited a psychologist and they tell them they are doing much better in their working lives with medication the psychologists have suggested that they may not need the medication any longer.'

'So the psychologists just see a higher form of positive emotion within their dialogue, just like a child perhaps,' said Mo.

'Indeed. It is also very important for employers to realise that only a small percent of any population have ADHD.'

'Which means that in most bigger organisations these people will be present and have a hard time,' said Mo.

'These employees will be mixed in amongst those people that really cannot be bothered.'

'But management cannot necessarily tell the difference. So the task-based problem rears its head again.'

'I'll give you an example when I worked for a clothing store. Every two months or so, we would get a return on an item.'

'So not a regular occurrence,' said Mo.

'I did not know how to refund a customer's money. One day, the boss of the shop told me I was stupid in front of the customer she was refunding the money to. She ushered me to one side with her hand, pressed a few keystrokes and completed the transaction.'

'But you had no way of recalling your past experiences to use in the present,' said Mo.

'I didn't have a clue. It was like I was looking at the keyboard for the first time. But it is simple to do, that's the point,' I said.

'So your bosses saw you couldn't do a job that honestly an eight-year old could do with their eyes closed.'

'I apologised for everything. I'd say it wouldn't happen again. The problem arose again but I couldn't justify my actions. The "three strikes out" in a job in Germany is commonplace.

'I would never be given more responsibility because I didn't gain the trust of the manager if I couldn't do simple tasks independently.'

'Which is reasonable.' said Mo.

'It is. I agree. But it isn't ever healthy for me!'

'But wasn't one of your earliest memories from when you were eight years old?' Mo asked.

'Yeah. I wrote in a diary when I was in Cornwall, England, in 1984 that everything was distracting me. And to this day, I haven't forgotten that'.

I even drew a picture that I have kept since that time.

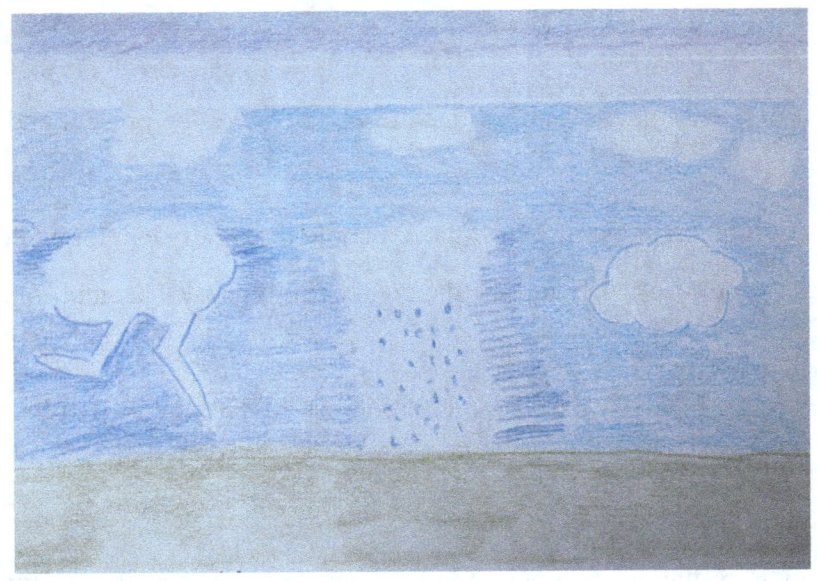

'What does it mean?' asked Mo.

'When I was eight years old, I decided that I didn't want a life full of bad weather, I wanted to be soaring where the peace and quiet was.'

'You knew at this age?' asked Mo.

'Yes, I did. But I didn't know how to get out of the bad weather I was in. I was eight. I had the firm belief that one day I would get out of the storm. I had nothing but belief and faith, (when I knew what faith meant) and would draw this picture at least once a year up until to-day. The picture in this book is from 2020.'

'Well you waited a long time!' said Mo.

'I waited over 30 years,'

'Is that why you have read self-development books for so long?'

'I guess so Mo. I found comfort in them. I believed I would find the solution and I didn't care how long it took.'

'So you were basically finding a solution to ADHD from a very young age?'

'I guess so,' I said to Mo.

'One day, I came across, in my opinion, the best self-development book ever.'

'What was that called?'.

'*Think and Grow Rich*, by Napoleon Hill. I must have read it over 100 times,' I said.

'But understood it about five times!' said Mo laughing.

'Yeah, probably I said,' laughing back.

'Why are you laughing?' asked Mo.

'I've just discovered the number one success principle that eclipses everything.'

'Which is?' said Mo, excited.

'I made it Mo. I now live my life in the thin white passage in the sky called clarity. I left the bad weather of distraction. This is what I always wanted since I was eight. Belief is the number one strategy.'

'But I can do something too!' said Mo.

'What then?' I ask.

'As I am also a part of you, I can now lay a hand on the head of my eight-year-old self and say "You don't have to worry anymore".'

'Thanks Mo,' I said.

Principles

- Life brings with it good and bad relationships. That is normal.

- Try to see which people in your life make you feel good and bad.

- Spend the least amount of time (none if possible) with those on your bad list but be polite and don't expect them to understand you if they aren't open to you! Keep the good people in your life and make life even greater with them!

- Dealing with ADHD is always a personal battle. I suggested that my wife leave me and find someone else without ADHD. I found that to be an absolutely normal phase that lasted for the first three months after the diagnosis, and while on medication. After that I haven't said it again!

- Your secure rating can only go up from now on. Get a copy of the book *Attached* and see what you think.

- The new you can improve existing relationships. You could fall in love with the person you married again.

- The 'full stop' phase. I had to see situations and people as they were over a period of a few weeks to have better judgement.

- Outsiders see an improvement of productivity and effectiveness in people that have ADHD and use medication. However, we need medication on a daily basis and for the rest of our lives. Our lives fall apart the instant we stop using medication.

- My first acknowledgement in the form of a picture and the word 'distraction' at the age of eight shows that it is possible to know at a young age that you have difficulties.

- From the age of eight years old I used belief, and faith (when I knew what that word was) knowing that this 'distraction' would one day disappear.

- The book *Think and Grow Rich* helped me understand how to best use belief and faith as an adult.

Chapter Eleven – My ADHD success meet-up group

'You put the word *success* in the name of your meet-up group?' Mo asked.

'I did!' I replied. 'People with ADHD can become highly successful,'

'Well, how are you going to promote that?' asked Mo.

'Stay calm and I'll tell you,' I smiled.

I launched my ADHD meet-up success group in September 2020 with the firm belief that, when dealt with intelligently, adults with ADHD in the community can make a really good life for themselves in all areas.'

'And you didn't want to come over as a phoney,' said Mo.

'Well, that is why I wrote this book.'

'Running a meet-up group gives me a sense of pride. I knew I would have no credibility for the first few years but I do have ADHD and can work from my own perspective. If I stand my reputation on the book I published, that is a good start. My book brings my success strategies with ADHD to a wider audience.'

'Boy does the world need to support this area a lot more,' said Mo.

'That is why I am doing it,' I said.

'Particularly with the success group, the *only* people who are interested in this area will turn up,' continued Mo. 'The ADHD success group started during the time of the coronavirus pandemic, right?'

'Yes, I would organise a meeting in the hope that we could meet,' I replied.

'Why didn't you do online conversations?' asked Mo.

'Because I felt it was important to meet face to face with the members to build up a social relationship,' I replied. The first couple of meetings would give the chance for people to get to know each other. I chose the first meeting to be held in a "family pub" environment instead of a self-help centre.'

'So everyone could relax?' asked Mo.

'Yes,' I replied.

'But the issues you bring up are very sensitive.' he added.

'Yes, I know, but a group has to start somewhere. I just think the added noises in our environment do help a little. I didn't want us to all talk in utter silence! I go and look at every venue before I organise something.

'The meeting starts with a quick introduction and then we would discuss which topic of interest we would like to be more *successful* at.'

'Are you making it fun?' said Mo.

'Yes. I would see which topic gets the most interest over ten-minute period. I give each member a pen and notepad so we can jot things down as we go. I do this because we have the tendency to write a lot about a subject. We are our own masterclass group in a way. We can hit a topic from all areas and then decide on what we need to concentrate on for the next four weeks.'

'The worst thing you can do to someone with ADHD is to take their notepad away,' said Mo laughing.

'You don't want to see what happens if you did that!' I said laughing back. 'The session is capped at an hour. I give them an assignment to complete within four weeks. This could be as simple as using the six-minute timer rule in a social setting and reporting back to be me with ten positives and two areas for improvement.'

'Why ten and two?' asked Mo.

'Because this is a success group Mo,' I replied. 'We concentrate on what works. I love this group and being around people.'

For so long, I felt I was the person Carl Gustav Jung, a Swiss psychiatrist and psychoanalyst was writing about: "Loneliness does not come from having no people about one, but from being unable to communicate the things that seem important to oneself, or from holding certain views which others find inadmissible." (Yung: 1963,P 356)

The group message is:

"We choose to make intelligent decisions in our lives by implementing strategies thought up in a group environment that bring us success. We will continue to learn   and in doing so pass on these positive messages so that everyone in this world can   benefit."

The group has been running for a year now and regular members benefit from this mutual understanding and success strategies they can implement in their lives.

'We can even revisit areas that were successful and tweak them to be better.'

'Why didn't you want to run the course in a conventional way?' asked Mo.

'I experienced a self-help group for ADHD first-hand. I quickly realised that the whole session revolved around negative life examples but rarely gave any solutions to the problems people were facing.

'Russell Barkley suggests "Avoid talk- or insight-orientated therapy, psychoanalysis, weekly group therapy focusing on complaining…". (2010: 93)'I mentioned before how I was working on improving on running an ADHD group successfully five years before even being diagnosed. I also knew that so many people in the population have ADHD but are not diagnosed. It took me ages to work out why if I have ADHD, I cannot independently come to a conclusion that my brain is malfunctioning because I use my own brain to come to that assumption in the first place.'

'So how did you go for an ADHD diagnosis in the first place?' asked Mo.

'I came back from a day at physiotherapy school in Berlin when my wife gave me a sheet of paper about specific traits that people with ADHD have.'

'And what did you do?'

'I took it to the bedroom and looked through it.'

My wife was sure that I had ADHD.

From her point of view, I had *all* of the points on the list of twenty things found with people who have ADHD, but thought it best not to say anything.

'I thought I had at least eleven of the traits on the list and I asked her help me find a doctor to diagnose me.'

After writing thirty letters to doctors in Berlin specialising in diagnosing adult ADHD, I was accepted for diagnosis testing at the Vivantes Clinic in Berlin.

'I went for checks over an eight-month period. I had medical checks on my heart, a random drug test, written tests of various kinds, had to speak openly about not fitting at school and being slandered regularly by my peers.'

'That's a lot.' said Mo.

'I was knackered after each session,' I replied.

'I had to write to my primary school in England to get a copy of any examination grades.'

'Which is really difficult because that was forty-two years ago,' said Mo.

'I then submitted all secondary school examinations to prove my grades were substandard.'

'This is why adults who think they have ADHD need to get a diagnosis done sooner than later?'

'Yes, because naturally some records will no longer be available,' I replied.

'So, it wasn't just a matter of turning up for a few checks at the hospital and hey presto, you have ADHD?'

'Not at all. I also had to complete an assessment review. When I was with my doctor, we had a telephone conference with both my parents. She took notes about my family history, how I behaved as a child, asked about school and friends to get a better picture of my life.'

'Which is difficult to do when someone is your age or older because some parents could be deceased,' said Mo.

'Exactly,' I said.

'But also, my parents spoke English of course.'

'Luckily your doctor spoke English,' said Mo.

'I know, it is presumed that German people can naturally speak English but not all of them can to a good level.

'I received the diagnosis on 2nd December 2019. The next day I saw my doctor who officially wrote on a document that I could be given ADHD medication pending a successful cardiac stress test.'

'So it wasn't as easy as getting the diagnosis and then medication?' said Mo.

'No, not at all. But I passed the tests and then had to find a doctor of psychiatry to give me a prescription for medication. That took a further four weeks to organise.

'I think the best route for an ADHD diagnosis is to go through a reputable organisation.

'But even during the testing phase you knew you had to get the word out.'

'I decided I had to write a book within the first year if I was ever diagnosed. I know there are people out there who are at their wits end, like me. I attended an ADHD self-help group because I wanted support during the diagnosis phase.'

'Which is totally fair enough,' said Mo.

'One night, while attending an ADHD self-help group, I heard a story from a father whose son has ADHD. I could feel his pain of living his life with a son he couldn't for some reason understand.

When I got home, I ran to the bathroom and was sick in the sink. I knew I could make a difference. After wiping my mouth, I made the following notes:

- Emphasis on strengths and not weaknesses.

- Individuals and families are at their wits end.

  1. Get the father and adult son to attend my group.

  2. They choose one area of their life to work on.

  3. Implement a success strategy gained from involvement from the whole group (more minds are better then one!).

4. They work on it for 4 weeks and explain the findings to the group focusing on success.

5. They implement this strategy into their lives.

'I then imagined every night for a week how I would run an ADHD differently. I came up with these suggestions.

- People need to understand this group is a *safe zone*.
- Their version of *Mo* can be present. It is unexpected and that this relationship with yourself can be a great one.
- I look forward to seeing the group come back with their findings a month later. Implementation of success strategies are fun! We can continue to use these.
  Seeing tangible results increases self-esteem.
- I see the beginning of awesome success stories coming to life.
- I thought being highly motivated was enough. It wasn't. I had a half-functioning motor until now. The motivation I had wasn't combined with self-confidence and this will probably be signalled in the demeanour of the members. Read into this.
- It doesn't matter at what age you get diagnosed. The diagnosis counts. Your future will be so much better than your past.
- Although it is very easy to feel victimised because you take medication, it is still your duty to make the best of your life and others because of chemical assistance.
- Having ADHD doesn't mean you are always the problem.
- I understand that there are many different people with ADHD. Some will take medication and some won't. I am unbiased. People need to do what they think is right.

'How did the first session of the success group go?' asked Mo.
'Well, of course I was nervous but I had the overriding feeling that what I was doing felt right.'
I introduced myself last one cosy evening at the restaurant, reading from a card I had prepared two months before.

My name is Simon and I have always believed that I could reach any goal I set for myself. I did everything I ever could to become a certified physiotherapist. I even studied this area in three different countries. But I didn't pass.

If you have ADHD everything in your foreground is distracting you. There was no way to get through the 95% of bedlam in your environment to use the last 5% of the concentration you have for a decent life.

I know, to a certain degree what everyone here is going through! I was diagnosed in 2019 with ADHD and take medication. I am however completely unbiased when it comes to people with ADHD using medication or not.

When sounds and distractions are removed in our world you are on a level playing field. I see a mixture of ages here today, some of you are in your twenties, some my age and some are older than me. I could imagine that many of you have had a really good shot at things in life which haven't come to fruition.

I guess that is why, in part, you are here today. To find the answers.

In this success group, we choose a topic of interest. We collaborate our ideas, come up with success strategies and report back to the group. I am just the mediator. I want a better life for adults with ADHD.

I'm here to remind you of the fire in your belly. It is still there. I had to push. You had to push.

But pushing never works.

The 95 percent distraction for many of us has now gone. The journey you need to succeed needs only 5 percent of your energy. Remind yourself of this every day.

There are no obstacles

Success will come to so much faster now...

So let's get going!

'In March 2021, I still only had five members. It is important that the members have been diagnosed with ADHD or are going for testing. I need to know that.'

'Why is this important?' said Mo.

'Because people with ADHD are a specific group. This book you have in your hands can be read by everyone but is directed at people who have ADHD themselves, those who think they have it and for those going for a diagnosis.

'At the very first meeting, in which everyone got to know each other, one of members suggested I hold an active meeting. We all live in the mountains and everyone thought it would be a great idea to go on a hike.'

Principles

– When dealt with intelligently, people with ADHD can become highly successful. Join or start a group that you find interesting to add value to people's lives with ADHD. A masterclass is a great source of help, inspiration, a common cause, friendship building and working together to improve our lives.

- Completing an assignment agreed on by the group to complete within four weeks. This could be as simple as using the six-minute timer rule in a social setting and reporting back with ten positives and two areas for improvement.

- Carl Gustav Jung, a Swiss psychiatrist and psychoanalyst was writing about loneliness when he said:

"Loneliness does not come from having no people around you, but from being unable to communicate the things that seem important to you". My group solves this!

- If I have ADHD, I cannot independently know that my brain is malfunctioning because I use my own brain to come to that assumption in the first place.

- People need to understand this group is a *safe zone*.

- Their version of *Mo* can be present. It is unexpected and that this relationship with yourself can be a great one.

- I look forward to seeing the group come back with their findings a month later. Implementation of success strategies are fun! We can continue to use these!
Seeing tangible results increases self-esteem!

- I see the beginning of awesome success stories coming to life.

- I thought being highly motivated was enough. It wasn't. I had a half-functioning motor until now. The motivation I had wasn't combined with self-confidence and this will probably be signalled in the demeanour of the members. Read into this.

- It doesn't matter at what age you get diagnosed. The diagnosis counts. Your future will be so much better than your past.

- Although it is very easy to feel victimised because you take medication it is still your duty to make the best of your life and others because of chemical assistance.

- Having ADHD doesn't mean you are always the problem.

- I understand that there are many different people with ADHD. Some will take medication and some won't. I am unbiased. People need to do what they think is right.

Chapter Twelve – The mountainous adventure

All of the members of the group met me in a town called Immenstadt on a Saturday morning in April. It was 18 degrees and sunny. The hike would lead us over a few peaks of the Nagelflukette mountain range. When everyone was ready, we started out from Marienplatz, the town square. Passing a sticky tape factory, we reached the Nagelfluhkette within ten minutes. Under our feet, the route changed from tarmac to soft woodland.

'This looks wonderful' said Maddie, the first person to sign up to the group.

We were immediately surrounded by waterfalls, rare alpine flowers and trees.

'This is a natural playground for us,' said Mereike.

Laughing could be heard from all around. We were standing in a protected national park that covers 405 thousand square metres. With ADHD, life can be tediously boring so something like a mountain is always welcome.

'Not only can you take the ski lift up to the top of my home mountain, you have the chance to hike up under your own ADHD steam!' said Mo. I acknowledged his presence with a smile.

We made our way upwards passing a sign advertising fresh cheese and milk at an alpine hut which would have opened us up to meadows and the route to the Mittagberg mountain, but we decided to follow the waterfalls instead.

We were all chatting away. I was getting bleeps from my iPhone every six minutes to remind me to let someone else speak in the group so I didn't get carried away.

Mike cheered us up even more by telling us a story as we walked through mist and water droplets. He said, 'Last year my family and I were hiking at the Silberklar gorge in Austria. There is a hut at the top of the mountain which we were heading for to have lunch.

'My kids and I would be looking at every single plant, tree, animal, climbing route and stone we could find. I didn't have medication then but crossing over a dry river bed was the best part. We looked at how the river bed was made up, we sorted odd pieces of bark from smallest to largest in a line wondering where they had come from. My wife was standing there rolling her eyes but we were busy and happy.

'It's funny how other people just tended to walk past us in the wrong kind of clothes such as jeans and a shirt while holding a bottle of coke in their hand walking like they have a plan to stick to, to get to the mountain hut, to not take in nature and its wonders. To express route everything!'

But then it started to rain – heavily! We got to the hut which was overflowing with people and managed to find a table. We were seated for an hour and a half. That was terrible. Within two seconds I got impatient when other people around me were relaxed. I couldn't understand why. Anyhow, we descended the mountain side once the rain had subsided. After walking for just ten minutes, we come across a group of about fifty people standing close together with panicked looks on their faces.

'I overhear one lady say, "We will never get out of here, the river is going to burst its banks." But it really was! The river was full! There was water rushing down the slope so fast that it would hit the top sides and smash over the bank. What a brilliant thing to see!! Jonathan, my oldest son and I split off immediately from the main group. My wife and younger son stood with the others. Jonathan gave me instructions to find a long plank of wood we had found earlier. I asked him where it was.

'"I threw it somewhere along here on the river bank," he said.

'Looking through the high grass, like lions observing gazelle, we found the plank twenty metres away. "Where did you find this?" I asked Jonathan, impressed. "Oh, I found this by those rocks over there earlier today," he said struggling with the ten-metre plank as my eyes opened with wonder and astonishment.

'I helped him pick up the plank, lay it over the stream which was about five metres wide, so not big enough to jump – and slowly one by one the group of fifty people saw we had a solution and crossed over to the other side. Not one person showed their appreciation. We were happy, but everyone was frantic. Within ten minutes, the people had completely disappeared. My son and I inspected more fauna amongst the rocks and river, which was now full. Johnathan looked at me while stroking the petals of a plant. He asked, "Why did the people just stand there like sheep when it is time to make a decision and get on with it?" I couldn't give him an answer. Sometimes not giving an answer is okay. But it got me thinking: how can society do well together and get jobs at work done properly but them fall into a panic when they have to act spontaneously? Why do normal people tend to stick together? At the hut everyone was warm and cosy and, happy, except us! Did they feel safe at the hut? I didn't. It's a strange phenomenon. It's like being part of society, but not really.

'With ADHD I guess every single mistake for us is level ten on the panic level. Do we just feel too much? I think we actually do. But we save the day when it comes to it! If we hadn't intervened I wouldn't know what would have happened. My best guess would be that the people would have waited it out. But it was still raining hard! Those people in trainers and t-shirts were not prepared at all! Would they have waited there until nightfall? I couldn't be sure!'

'That's a great story,' I said.

'Your son was the hero of the day,' commented Mereike.

'After the holiday in Austria, my son and I would talk often about the river experience. It was fun. It is something we will never forget'. Mike finished.

So, we continue hiking with the group and enter a coniferous tree zone. The smell is amazing. Everything around us looked different. Any chance to see an endangered butterfly called the Apollofalte or a rare hen called the Auerhuhn, also called a *Standvogel* because it lives in the same area all year round kept our brains in gear.

Then, from out of nowhere, a tractor comes whizzing down the path we are walking on. Mike crumbles down a small embankment.

We were all surprised because we have a tendency to hyper-focus on individual things. We didn't even see Mike disappear.

'Good job you let out a cry,' I said, lending him a hand.

'Otherwise, I would have been there for a long time.' he joked.

'Yeah, probably,' I replied.

We pulled Mike up onto his feet and I asked him if he lost his balance often.

'No,' he replied, 'but the tractor did a good job!' he said laughing.

As the sun was warming our fronts, I got talking to another member of the group called Jessica, who originally comes from Poland. Her spoken German was very good so I complimented her on it. She thanked me for the comment and said that many people would say that her German is good but she never wanted their standard as her goal post. I asked her why she thought that way.

She said 'People just see a snapshot, a moment! I first noticed when I was doing well at German when I realised it myself. I once went to a Scrabble class in Berlin and lasted two sessions. I wasn't any good but that wasn't due to ADHD!'

'It must have been an interesting experience,' I said.

'I played a couple of games when I was there. The members told me I was as good as any German person. I got 300 points and only had lived in the country for 3 months. I thought it would be cool thing to try out.'

'That is pretty good,' I replied.

'Well, I played Scrabble quite a lot as a kid,' she said.

'What did your opponent get?' I asked.

'Oh, he got like 720 points.'

'Wow!' I said 'I didn't know you could get that many points.'

'Neither did I,' she replied 'but the group was getting in hours of practice before they went to the world championships.' she giggled.

'I can see why they let you go,' I giggled back.

'Yeah, so although I have my ADHD it isn't like I'm not clever. I just think I am pretty average,'

'I agree,' said Maddie.

'I think we are very fortunate to use our brains differently now than we used to. It doesn't necessarily mean that we are superhuman or better than everyone else. I think we have just been bought into line with our environment. We are learning new things, I guess like kids do, and we are enthusiastic about that'.

After three hours into our hike, we reached the furthest point from Immenstadt. It was time to head back, taking a different route. A route with covered with snow. We couldn't see the path under our feet but my GPS showed us a virtual path perfectly. It didn't stop Mereike getting her feet stuck, in which Mike for the second time held her upright to stop the shoe coming off as she took another step.

Later on, we were dragging each other through bogs. Jessica fell onto her back so I pulled her up. We stood there for a minute and she went quiet. I asked her if everything was ok.

She replied 'Simon, I have never seen anyone so hands on as you.'

'I was just pulling you up,' I said a little surprised.

'But you did it with energy and finesse, you didn't want to let me go,'

'I wanted you to get out of the mud,' I replied 'that's all.'

I admitted it wasn't the first time someone has told me I am too hands on.

'You know why that is.' said Mo.

'No,' I said aloud while everyone was looking at me strangely.

'It means you are that person who will drop everything there and then to help someone out,'

'Oh, thanks,' I replied.

I wanted to discuss this topic with the group to see what they had to say about people being too hands on.

Mereike said that she sees it too in herself. 'I know that I need an increased amount of touch in my life as well as my daughter who also has ADHD. There is a lady who organises horse riding lessons in the Allgäu for kids with ADHD purely to increase the sense of touch.'

'That sounds great,' said Mike.

'But an increased need of touch in society is deemed inappropriate,' Mereike said.

'But look at it another way,' said Tom interrupting. 'I have kids too and they have access to weighted blankets, and that is a form of touch, or in other words, security. But look at what we have done today in the form of security,' he continued. 'As a group, we enjoyed dipping our feet into the stream from the waterfall and it felt great. We increased group and individual security. Individual touch is running your hand through leaves on the trees. All of us here have lived lifetimes just in the present tense. We lived in the moment, we have lived each moment and it is wonderful! Touch is an immediate sense.'

The afternoon was really good fun. Some of the group bought fresh cheese from a vending machine, on the mountain! We even had to ascend a cliff face using a metal chain to guide ourselves. We were quiet, we were loud but most of all we got to know each other.

The hike took seven hours. We got back to Immenstadt, some had a quick coffee and then got in their cars to drive home. A couple of them enjoyed looking at the scenery one more time before the light faded for the day. When everyone had gone, I reached into my backpack, which always houses a notepad and pen and wrote the following:

ADHD people are amazing!!

I truly think that people with ADHD bring our world not just joy and happiness but could change how workforces operate and how things can be done differently. It is probably more difficult for people with ADHD who have decided not to take medication to lead a good life but there are those that do it, and do it well.

Many people are not diagnosed due to many reasons and those who are and take medication also see improvements in their lives. I appreciated this today in hearing the stories that were said. We are the people that are constantly on the corners of society. We have a quintessential character trait of just getting up and carrying on. If you are like me and have a soft loving personality this can be seen negatively, although everyone at some basic level needs belonging and to be liked. Perhaps people are not willing to admit it, like we are.

Perhaps we are just seen as the people who cannot show our teeth, make a strong decision or lead a team. In truth we know ourselves better than most, from the inside. That is where leadership of yourself and others start and we do it creatively and not by the book! I thoroughly enjoyed today's experience and look forward to another adventure soon.

Principles

- The wonders of nature help all people and those with ADHD to increase the quality of life.
- Hiking up a mountain under your own ADHD steam is wonderful – try it.
- People with ADHD can be very good in stressful situations.
- You know you are good at something when you realise it yourself.
- People with ADHD can be bought into line with their environment. They can be deemed as very clever. Naturally people with ADHD will fall into all levels of intelligence. But our brains work differently, which gives us a good edge in life.
- People with ADHD need an increased amount of touch in their lives which society deems inappropriate. Touch can also include shaped benches for sitting on at the dinner table, embossed cushions or even weighted blankets.
- People with ADHD know themselves better than most, from the inside.

Chapter Thirteen – How sporting environments bring out my best ideas

One day, I decided to go out to a local town to enjoy a cup of tea and a nice piece of cake. I ended up in Kempten, where I regularly run my meet-up group but this time I just wanted to ponder some ideas.

As I sat down to a table I glanced through the window and saw a picture of a fitness nutrition shop with a man and women in an advert looking very trim with their six packs.

'You had a six pack once,' said Mo.

'I had a very flat stomach,' I replied.

'You starved me to death doing that,' he commented.

'No, of course not,' I replied. 'But seriously, I learnt so much from that time. 'In 2017 I wanted to get really fit. I wanted to get a six pack for the first time in my life. I knew I had to eat less and train hard but I needed pressure from the outside too. I had undiagnosed ADHD and wanted some real excitement in my life! I found the idea of putting myself into a realm that others couldn't understand or follow very interesting. So, I told people at work that "in twelve weeks I will be standing in front of you, ready for summer with a six pack".'

'How did that go down?' Mo said.

'Like a lead balloon,' I replied. 'But that is what I wanted! I knew that this example could be achieved through *doing* and not *thinking*. I knew this is where my self-confidence sits. A strong body is the ground stone to fend of psychological attacks. A good-looking body is also on the extreme side of life that people are not comfortable with. But at that time, I wanted a six pack for summer, plain and simple. I joined the Sharny and Julius fit dad programme and arranged my sleeping, eating and training around the advice they gave. My kids saw the results and they loved it when I was lying on the floor chest pressing them.

'What?' said Mo impressed.

'I was doing kettle bell swings with them too! After exercise I felt good about myself.'

'That was cool getting the kids involved,' said Mo.

'It was Sharny and Julius's workout idea to get the kids involved! Anyway, people at work would see me losing weight and say it's not possible, you can't do it. I would reply "Yes, I can". I started at 18 per cent body fat and was dropping the fat fast. At 6 weeks in, I was getting fit. "Look at Simon, he thinks he can get a six pack." people were saying laughing in front of me. I kept saying to them "I can do this".'

'But it didn't get any easier,' said Mo. 'people got really rude and angry.'

'I was completing forty-five minutes of abdominal training every day. When I look back, I think it was the best thing I could have done with undiagnosed ADHD. At the end of July, I was eating a snack during break time when a colleague said "You didn't get the six pack, then?". I immediately pulled up my t-shirt, showed him my flat stomach and he went quiet. I had made it!

'I was at eleven percent body fat and dropped from seventy-eight to seventy kilograms. I was lean and I knew it. I didn't have the six pack because I would have had to drop lots more body fat than that but I had a flat stomach which was good enough. Then an amazing thing happened.

'This colleague of mine told everyone else and the news spread like wildfire. Within half a day, everyone wanted to see the results. They were proud of me. I was holding the flag. I had positively influenced my colleagues by completing this challenge, and I liked it.

'People just need to be shown the way. And this is how I operate in my life now, due to this one success. This success burned something very positive into me. I knew it had to be reciprocal in other areas of my life.'

'And at some point, you went to work in a fitness club,' said Mo.

'That's right,' I said. 'I was going through the diagnosis for ADHD when I first started working there. A family friend suggested I go and speak with the manager and he liked what I said and employed me the following week.'

'You loved working at that club.'

'I really did,' I said.

Let me explain it a little further.

Principles

- Achieve one single goal that you can reach from doing and not thinking. A fitness goals are a good example. I achieved this with undiagnosed ADHD. I found the idea of putting myself into a realm that others couldn't understand or follow very interesting.
- A strong body can fend off psychological attacks.
- Stage 1 of achievement of a goal – People will ridicule you if this goal is on the extreme side of life.
- Stage 2 – Then people get rude and angry.

- Stage 3 – I achieved my goal. Others were proud of me. I was holding the flag. I had positively influenced my colleagues by completing this challenge, and I liked it.
- You only need one success to give you a burning desire in its achievement to propel you forward in life and to reflect on those moments when times are hard. You become unstoppable!

Chapter Fourteen – The fitness club

I had started working at a fitness company straight after I failed the physiotherapy course, before being diagnosed with ADHD. I kept this information very quiet. After all, I might not get a positive diagnosis (which you, the reader, have to keep in mind if you are going for testing).

I noticed straight away that I was in a very caring environment. I was learning the ropes and found that checking members in or out while also taking phone calls hard to manage. Not a good first impression! But doing the job I was employed to do on the fitness floor wasn't that easy either. Compiling fitness plans was straightforward but I couldn't type into the computer the three actions required in sequence to start a VO_2 max fitness test, even though I was doing this nearly every single day.

After three months, those three steps should have been natural. They weren't. I felt stupid. Fortunately, my two bosses planned feedback meetings into the work schedule. Every three weeks, we would talk about my progress. These were great meetings. I would get honest feedback. I would hear what I was doing wrong but they gave me ideas on how to improve. When a meeting was forthcoming, I found it helpful to ask if the meeting would be a *good* or a *bad* one. I couldn't understand social and work related clues very well but I guess, likewise, they probably had difficulty understanding me too. I had experienced many bad meetings when working in Berlin. I would prepare documents ready to submit to the unemployment office the night before a meeting, just in case I lost my job. I got quite good at the process. But that is no way to live.

'I know why you think this way in the first place,' said Mo.

'Ok, tell me,' I said to Mo.

'You were talking with a shop manager one day about how he chooses the people he employs. He said that people are chosen to work in a working environment due to their skill set.'

'Fair enough,' I said. 'He also said the following, "In my area, people are chosen for their command of English, confidence and their selling power. Fifty-five percent of people stay within certain behavioural boundaries, and fifteen percent change their behaviour entirely and get thrown out within a year."'

'And you didn't want to be thrown out of a company if they knew you had changed your behaviour?' said Mo.

'True, but I think people do have to adjust to their environment. No one stays the same, everyone changes,' I said.

'Yes, but the changes just shouldn't be too much in a positive or negative way as the bosses had got to know you in the first place,' said Mo.

'My bosses and I agreed at the first meeting that it would be a good idea if I can help colleagues of mine complete certain jobs when they were busy. They would give me the outline of what I had to do. I would write my own checklist. However, a simple distraction such as making a coffee for someone and then answering a ringing phone was close to impossible. Either the person on the end of the phone or the member waiting too long for their coffee wondered what is wrong most of the time. I was not giving good service. Ticking off the checklist was one important form of achievement. I needed my list!'

'I didn't realise you needed a check list that badly,' said Mo.

'I did. But it got a little strange, one day,' I replied. 'One of my bosses wondered if I worked on a *trial and error* system. I asked her what she meant. She said to me, "The daily operations of the club are similar every single day. Which means they don't change much. It should be simple for you to do after a while. I have never met someone like you before. It's like you are born into each day fresh, naive, innocent."'

'How did you respond to that?' asked Mo.

'I thought she was pulling my leg,' I replied. 'But then I realised I work in Germany!'

'Got it,' said Mo.

'I knew what she meant but not in its entirety. We both couldn't put our thumb on it. I couldn't yet bind one job in a certain time zone with the next job that came up in the future. It was like the mesh wasn't holding things together. My whole life was in fact a puzzle. I would still not know how to do the 'basics' of my job. In Germany, the work ethic is very strong but I couldn't tell the difference between doing a good job and 'perfectionism'.'

I knew this but just wanted to offer a good service in an area that I am good at, and that was in fitness. So, with the tasks I had at work I had to seriously chunk everything down. I had, up until now been getting things done as fast as possible. Now I can let a moment 'hang' in the air. I hadn't seen the possibility of seeing a whole day in front of me before. I can now have an official break without burning myself out or wondering anymore if, in fact, I could get all of the jobs done that I said I would. Before my diagnosis I was doing 'excessive reaching' for everything.

'After I was diagnosed, I distinctly thought long and hard as to whether I should tell my employer or not. I decided that I would. These are great people. I had to tell them. So, I did and it was as shocking for them as it was for me. I told them I would take medication but needed time to get the right dose. It took, I think about two months to fine tune this.'

'Then your work life picked up, I can remember,' said Mo.

'I was getting all of my jobs done, I could tell if a job was urgent or not when I couldn't before.'

'I even remember you doing things without people asking and they would be surprised,' finished Mo.

'Yeah, I loved completing an extra job because I actually had time left over!'

'But the relationships I had with everyone started to fail, Mo.' I said in a sad tone. 'On one hand I could design a fitness programme better than before. The members were elated. I was using such a broad range of exercises, some had never seen before. But I noticed I was focusing my eyes on what was in front of me instead of what was happening peripherally. I would have a member on the telephone wanting to attend a class and I would be inputting their details into the computer. Meanwhile another member arrives or leaves the club on foot. I wouldn't see the member leaving because all I saw was the computer screen. I wouldn't say Hello or Goodbye, either.

I guess my bosses didn't really know what was going on. Heck, I didn't either. They both asked if I was having therapy.

'I told them I was looking forward to my first session.'

'Oh, I remember this,' said Mo.

'What, when I went for my initial appointment?' .

'Yes,' he said trying to contain himself.

'I thought it was a bit strange from the outset,' I said. 'The therapist spent more time looking in a text book because she didn't know what ADHD was and then cross referenced it with what I was saying to come to the conclusion that it all did add up' I said. 'That was annoying!'

'I loved that,' said Mo.

'What?' I replied.

'It was like a game of tennis' he said laughing, 'the eyes of the therapist were going from the book…to you…to the book…to you.'

'Ok, I get your point,' I said.

'Good joke,' Mo replied. 'You must have been thinking *she can't be serious*!' finished Mo, screaming with laughter.

'I was not impressed,' I finished.

'It served you right,' quipped Mo.

'Shut up, Mo,' I finished.

Going to work in a supportive environment, working with great colleagues and super members of the fitness club was a good reason to get up every day. But I felt I was being robbed of the old Simon.

It was already annoying having to go to therapy when therapists don't know what ADHD is!

'But in all honesty, Simon, said Mo, 'you can't expect therapists to know about every clinical subject in detail.'

'I agree,' I replied 'but isn't that the very point? If I couldn't get help in this very sensitive area, which I searched out actively because I needed answers, then I thought I could do this myself.'

'But you only had visited the *one* therapist,' replied Mo.

'I know that,' I replied. 'But from what I have heard, ADHD is the most researched mental illness out there. Wouldn't it be fair to assume that an internet search in a big city would bring up loads of therapists who specialise in adult ADHD?' I asked Mo.

'Not necessarily,' he replied.

'Why?' I asked.

'Because,the population who have ADHD is only between four to five percent, according to Dr Barkley,' he finished. (2010:2)

'But that alone would equate to around 180,000 people in Berlin having ADHD at five percent. I know many kids would have it but the number of adults is a huge number also. Listen, I know you have a good point Mo, but don't forget my world was completely turned upside down from one day to another.'

'So what did you do about it?' asked Mo.

'I started to exercise with ADHD to make me feel better. I realised loads of new things especially when I spoke to a close friend of mine.'

Principles

- Think about whether you want to tell your employer that you have ADHD. You don't have to.

- Routine jobs such as typing a sequence of key stokes into a computer to start a VO_2 max fitness test, even though I was doing this nearly every single day was very difficult. I could do this now with medication.

- Are you working on a trial and error system like my boss saw I was doing? Have you even noticed this in yourself? I couldn't yet bind one job in a certain time zone with the next job that came up in the future. If so, does this mean you don't know the 'basics' of your job.

- Seriously chunk everything down. I had, up until now been getting things done as fast as possible because I only knew the present! Now I can let a moment 'hang' in the air. I hadn't seen the possibility of seeing a whole day in front of me before. I can now have an official break without burning myself out or wondering anymore if, in fact, I could get all of the jobs done that I said I would.

- I felt for a long time that I was being robbed of the old Simon when I started on medication. The correct dosage can take at least a couple of months if not more. It is possible that you may change again throughout the years. I had a new personality immediately with the medication and it takes a long time to get used it. My strengths and weakness changed overnight. But life will work out just fine! That is why I have written this book!

- Don't be surprised if you can't find any psychotherapists specialising in adult ADHD. It may take a couple of goes until you find the correct person for you. Ask your therapist if they know what ADHD actually is! I now have a great therapist.

Chapter Fifteen – Sport and ADHD

A friend of mine admitted he runs twelve miles just to calm down. I did the same with cycling before I was diagnosed. On one particular week, he got to the eight-mile mark and was feeling good. At ten miles in, he ran out of energy. He had no food or drink on him. His called his mother to bring some coffee and drive him home. He had totally overestimated himself. We compared each others' experiences.

'In the past I would cycle forty kilometres before work to rid myself of the fidgeting inside of me. I couldn't cycle this distance every day just to calm down, but what other option did I have?' I told my friend.

'Cycle a shorter distance,' said Mo.

'A distance shorter than forty kilometres wouldn't work. I would still be fidgety. Not with arms flaring around kind of fidgety but more like my inner body was having a party without my brain's consent. My workouts were inconsistent. My friends were too.'

He told me he was going for ADHD diagnosis so I asked him to give me two weeks to compile an exercise success list from the experiences and notes I wrote over the last year. I would then send him my findings. I did it solely because I didn't want to get another phone hearing that he had got into trouble again.

Exercise – newly diagnosed with ADHD and taking medication – Month 1 to Month 4

– I took a month to get used medication. (No exercise).

- I worked for a fitness club. I joined a few classes. I was guided through the exercise. I didn't need to overthink what I was doing. On medication, I had enough to think about.

- My balance wasn't good over this period due to hyper-focus.

- I thought that medication would unlikely constitute a change in muscle length, strength or weakness.

- I found a training partner. We would complete floor-based activities and use resistance machines. I stayed away from dumbbells because of balance problems.

Note: In the past my friend and I both had fitness club memberships. However, we always missed the bus to get there, although we knew what time it would leave. If we got the bus on time, we were impatient with the thirty-minute commute. We both couldn't stand the loud music when we got there so ended up leaving early and going home.

'But you saw a solution after month four,' said Mo.

'I decided to work out at home!' I laughed.

Exercise – Month 4 and 5

- Because I am on constant release medication, I have experienced sometimes heavier releases of the drug into my system later in the day, which makes me a little annoying to be around. This only happens about once or twice a month. I tend to exercise in the morning to smooth this problem out. In these cases, I need to remind myself that things are okay. Have a quick 'check in' with myself.

- I bought an indoor rower. I could get a good workout in at any time! I was in the comfort of my own home. The kids would be in bed, all the lights would be off except for my rowing monitor and I would row 5km. I termed this 'midnight rowing'. Knocking out all my senses seemed to help. I have a notebook and pen next to me. I was filling up my inner world with good ideas and suggestions.

'But you were getting sore,' said Mo.

'And I finally had an answer for that,' I said.

- I purchased a small whiteboard. I would complete a workout and write on it the exercise and duration. I knew that muscle soreness lasts for up to seventy-two hours. For the next two days I had a visual prompt. I had calmness of mind. When the muscle soreness disappeared, I scrubbed the board clear and was ready for the next workout.

- When I was undiagnosed with ADHD but injured, I was given physiotherapy exercises. I kept all of these and now and use these as a blueprint for my training.

- When cycling I use a GPS with a timer. My body (when I take medication) gave me an indication when I was warm (for the first time in my life). This could take twenty to fifty minutes. I then would pick up speed for a while and then have a cool down phase of five kilometres. I found my heart rate decreased when I was cycling past cows by up to ten beats per minute. I now search out routes in the countryside and stay away from roads.

-       Nordic walking. Our legs are contact points to the ground but we have two additional contact points to the ground in form of sticks in our hands. With ADHD, we know that distractions are normal such as streams, animals and the ground we walk on, i.e. gravel, bark, grass and stone. We use our lower and upper body simultaneously. This helps with balance.

-       ADHD people probably have a tendency to do sport alone. When doing sport outside, take a small backpack with you. Include a charged phone, magnesium sachets to stop cramping, cola for a caffeine kick, water, extra clothes and muesli bar, tell someone where you are going and for how long. Take an identification card and a small amount of change (money) with you. I have a normal health insurance and a mountain rescue card. I have the tendency to increase exercise duration from what is planned. Just make sure you can get back home.

Exercise Month 6

By now, I had come across the ideal that ADHD is a really balance between the brain, the body and outside forces of life. I knew that core training to keep the stomach and back equally strong would be a good start.

'Then you joined a martial arts class,' said Mo.

'I thought my balance and coordination was worse on medication from the first day I started taking it. I thought it could improve this area.'

'You now love Kung Fu,' said Mo.

'I really do,' I replied. 'The people make the class. They are a really friendly bunch. When we do sequences it isn't the master who always comes to alter my body position but anyone in the group.'

'How good is that?' said Mo excited.

'It's brilliant. I learnt how to concentrate by using whole sight rather than just the hyper-focus.'

'Because blocks and strikes come at you from different angles?' asked Mo.

'Yes,' I replied 'I was re-learning spatial awareness.'

'You also needed to be fairly agile for meditation,' said Mo.

I had been meditating at least twice a week for a year leading up to my ADHD diagnosis and really enjoyed it. It would really calm me down and at some periods I would sit in the Lotus position for up to three hours and feel really refreshed afterwards.

'And then you spoke to an instructor at your work who runs meditation classes,' said Mo.

'That was a pretty interesting talk, actually,' I said. 'She told me many people have trouble with the phase leading into the depth of meditation, they find it uncomfortable and many cannot go any further. I said I find it very easy to slip into meditation, which got me thinking as to why. I came to the conclusion that with undiagnosed ADHD it's the only time I could actually shut down the world around me. Three hours of meditating is a long time and obviously my body needed it.'

'But your findings didn't stop there,' said Mo.

'The drop into meditation is in my opinion identical as dropping into medication,' I said.

'What do you mean?' said Mo.

'The phase of becoming quiet inside, more concentration, ignoring outside sounds is for me the same when meditating as when on my tablet. I thought that meditation could bring me into a meditative state that I could use when undiagnosed to succeed with my day.

But I could never have a successful day. My environment was as aloud as ever even after three hours sitting on my mat at home before I started my day. I actually tried it!'

'That's so bad!' said Mo.

Exercise Month 8

- I mountain biked through snow and ice for fifty-five kilometres. I didn't fall over once! I concluded that if my balance was affected by medication, I would fall around on a daily basis and I wasn't.

When I had the prior information finished, I sent the bullet points over to my friend. He had then been diagnosed with ADHD and was very pleased that he had at least some information as to what to expect with his first year of medication (which he opted for).

I wrote a few principles for him afterwards to help calm his mind and sent the following also to him.

Principles

- We were so focused on getting rid of our pent-up energy through sport. We can enjoy sport now.

- Let a fitness instructor write you a programme. You have to know when to let other people take over.

- Don't be embarrassed about taking medication.

- Find a training partner for friendship and accountability.

- Meditation is wonderful. I choose guided meditation in the evening when I come off my medication for the day.

- You can now plot muscle soreness. You couldn't remember before and that is okay! You will save time not going to doctor with every niggle.

- When you were out running and could feel your troubles running with you instead of disappearing you did this until you collapsed. I have done this too. That was a bad time. Know that medication can bring peace to your soul and this shouldn't happen again.

- If you are out running in a group, run your pace. When I ran fitness classes, I wanted to meet my clients' expectations but ignored my own. A general life rule: remember you cannot give more of what you don't have.

- When cycling, take a few water bottles with you. In the early days of using medication, I had to drink more water than normal because of a dry mouth.

'Did he like what you sent?' asked Mo.

'He loved it!' I said ecstatically. 'My friend was really humbled with the information I sent to him, purely because the information is so personal. He thought more people should know about this: that people in general need an update about ADHD. But my friend was having trouble with the changes in his new life, especially at night time. He only had me to talk to. He didn't know what was happening. He needed someone to talk to immediately instead of reading a book. So, to his relief I was at home when he called one night.'

'What did you talk about?'

'Well, fortunately I had written the chapter for this book, which describes the evening routine I use when coming off of my medication.'

'I bet he was pleased!' said Mo.

'Yeah, I guess I was his lifesaver that night,' I replied.' A person who doesn't have ADHD will not even begin to understand how bad our lives can be at night time after a recent diagnosis.'

'I went through the chapter with him (not the full chapter because his experience made me write even more for this section), which is entitled "The dark side of ADHD". Easing him into it gently giving him the reassurance that I understood his dilemma, that he could understand my point of view but starting with a pleasant story during day time, to relax him before I presented the more pressing issues of the evening.'

'Good idea,' said Mo.

'We spoke for over two hours and I answered any questions there and then. I then sent him an individual bulleted list the next day that he could immediately implement.'

'So tell us more!' said Mo.

'I'd love to,' I replied.

Chapter Sixteen – The dark side of ADHD (and how to deal with it!)

It took me ten months to become unstuck with a part of the ADHD puzzle, which I would like to share with you now.

I was sitting on a rock one day at our local lake in summer watching my sons playing with a ball five metres away from me. I noticed when the kids were further apart from each other I could only concentrate on one of them.

'So you were hyper-focusing,' said Mo.

'Yes. The kids were having so much fun but I felt very distant. I would see families around me relaxing, chatting and having fun. I was in my own bubble. I felt I was glued to the spot. But I felt comfortable inside this bubble but also felt like my life was in the shadows and is seeping by minute, by minute.

'I wondered how people would see me sitting there. Would they see emotions of loss and sadness? Would I be, in their eyes an approachable person? I didn't honestly have an answer.

'I felt I was losing my life more with medication.

'I felt I was losing reality and for a time I hated it.'

'But was that where the buck stopped?' asked Mo.

'I decided to make a positive turnaround.'

I knew that distractions in my environment were reduced significantly. What I was feeling for a long time was *myself.*

Before I was diagnosed, I said to someone that my two kids are really annoying. This guy asked me "Can't you just ignore them?" I looked at him and said 'I can never *ever* ignore them!'

I never have wanted to ignore my kids but I can sit and enjoy watching them playing among themselves. I can be *me.*

I also could differentiate between impulsivity (which I don't have now) and being 'overly keen'. The people I saw around me at the lake were strangers. I didn't know anyone, but I am a chatty person. So, instead of talking to strangers I decided to start an 'hour of enjoyment' with my kids. I used to go swimming in a fifty-metre pool on a Friday afternoon in Brisbane with the three dollars I had as disposable income in 2003 so I used this idea and took the kids to an outdoor pool ten minutes' walk from our home.

We had a great time, just the three of us! They even did some brainstorming on what else they wanted to do. We slowly built up our hour of enjoyment into a whole day of activities.

We hired a Stand-up paddle board and found peace and quiet in the middle of a lake. It was a great experience. I made sure I wasn't the dad who sat by himself on the rock. I was better than that.

'I guess the audiobook from John Maxwell you often listen to, *Winning is an Inside Job*, was starting to rub off on you?' said Mo.

'I was definitely now winning on the inside and people would gravitate to me. I now keep things very *locker*, (relaxed) as we say in German. I also have a mental check in with myself every hour, which is nice too.

'You were bringing excitement back into your life,' said Mo.

'I really was,' I replied. 'At night when I come off of medication, I wondered what was happening with my brain function.'

'A new topic to get your teeth into!' said Mo.

'Yes, I really wanted to understand the transition my brain was going through.'

I learnt from my prescribing doctor that when the medication wears off, I go into a negative swing where my ADHD symptoms are worse for a short period of time before I come back to my normal unmedicated ADHD state.

I knew that the medication I take works for thirteen hours. Fifteen minutes before the thirteen-hour mark I will find a quiet place and listen to guided meditation. I feel I need an hour to come back to normal. Listening to positive relaxing guided meditation with the lights off is something I can really recommend.

'That is a good solution,' said Mo.

'Yes, I said, it really is!'

'But there is a huge flaw when my medication wears off that I didn't realise until now.' I said.

'Which is?' asked Mo.

'This time of the day put the most stress on the relationship between myself and my wife. She admitted that this phase didn't deteriorate our relationship when I asked her about it though!'

'At least she could differentiate,' said Mo.

'"But it would completely ruin every evening with my boys!" she had said.'

'How so?' asked Mo.

'We could be watching a film and I would get up and leave to go to the bedroom for an hour to complete two guided meditation sessions.'

'That is still positive,' said Mo.

'On one side, I calm down. The process is quite odd and I do cry most nights for the first five minutes, which is why I choose guided meditation instead of doing it from my own perspective. But after about ten minutes I am very relaxed. After forty-five minutes I write everything down on paper.'

'Has it worked?' asked Mo.

'It has been an amazing experience. I have experienced things during meditation which I cannot explain. After the hour, I go back to the family and have a really positive attitude and sleep very well now every night. This information really helps my friend out now.

'I told him that during mediation once, I could smell a fragrance on someone I got to know in Australia almost twenty years ago.'

'Wow, what did you do?'

'I looked online as to what it could be. Found a bottle that looked like it could be the right one, not having seen the packaging before and went to my local store the next day.'

'And…?' said Mo.

'They had the perfume. I knew it was the right one. I grabbed one of those paper strips they have to spray the scent on and did that.'

'And…?' said Mo again.

'It was the fragrance!'

'Wow,' said Mo.

'Yeah, I felt like I was taken back in time.'

'But I went a step further,' I added. 'I bought the perfume and sent it to the lady. I felt amazing for doing that!'

'I bet you did.'

'The first sign of knowing that I am coming off of the medication is that I look around for something for half an hour. This is most often my iPod with the meditation mp3 on it. This not knowing where something is very annoying and this happens a few times a week because I meditate in different places. Which means I stay up longer at night which decreases the amount of sleep I actually get. This is dependent on whether I actually find the iPod. Remember, I have to get up early to take my medication which takes an hour to start working in my body. Only then am I concentrated for thirteen consecutive hours. I cannot, during these hours sit down and relax. I am concentrating for the whole duration. Therefore, you can see that if I take my medication at 5.30 am, it starts to work at 6.30am until 7.30 pm. I then have the coming-off process of an hour and I do like to spend the evening with my wife and kids after all.

'This is why I have to keep things as tidy as possible. I'm not a minimalist but less stuff equals less stress. I have to know where everything is!

'During the first year, I used to go for a walk outside at night at the thirteen-hour point. I didn't take anything with me apart from a small 'Hundert Wasser' notepad and pen. If I was unlucky, when I got back, I ended up shouting at my wife. She realised this is a result of coming off the medication and she dealt with by not dealing with me.'

A prime example of this is from *The Chronicles from the Future*:

"People tell each other how they feel and whatever the outcome – acceptance or separation – they have told the truth. In fact, most of the time, acts such as these are forgiven, especially if it's an infatuation, a moment of passion or a loss of self-control" (Dienach. 129/130).

'It is good that your wife is so understanding.' said Mo.

'I agree,' I said. 'In the evening, I have the option of guided meditation, herbal teas, stretching and drawing and visualising techniques. Please understand that it is the realisation within yourself that brings about new and positive changes in your life. You can only do that, I think when you know yourself completely.

'My friend asked me if I had ever not taken medication the next day to see how it goes.'

'Totally relevant,' said Mo. 'I guess he wanted to know of the medication can work for a longer period of time, for example days or weeks.'

'He didn't want to go through the coming-off phase every day, and I get it, it's isn't nice. I told him that I didn't take medication one morning and started working through my check list for the day. I didn't know what I was looking at and I couldn't complete tasks to the end. Every attempt even broken down to half an hour slots, then fifteen-minute slots, even five-minute slots wouldn't work. I went from one thing to another wondering how I got there. I was impulsive again. That's the tiring part.

'The next day (so the second day of not taking medication in a row), I summoned up even more motivation and even did meditation to bring me into line but after half of the second day there were still loose ends, I couldn't understand important emails that were in my inbox. I was exhausted by the time midday came around.'

'But you noticed something very key fifteen months after your diagnosis!'

'Thanks for reminding me Mo,' I said. 'Off of medication on the second consecutive day, I realised you were completely gone Mo. The voice of anxiety chips in quietly again. I realised this terrible little voice was back.'

'Terrible?' said Mo.

'Terrible and small,' I replied. 'Because I read motivational books and listen to audio recordings every day, I will always feel a voice of one of them talking to me. One night, I had Lisa Nichols come to me saying she would look after me through the night until Mo comes backs in the morning.'

'That's a bit far out,' said Mo.

'I guess these mentors of mine, such a Bob Proctor (my number 1) are so embedded in my daily life I feel the positive energy from their messages – and it works! I concluded that I have to live every day of my life with medication. I knew I am not going to one day wake up normal,' I replied.

'Does that worry you?' asked Mo.

'Do you know what worries me the most Mo?' I said with sadness.

'What is it Simon, you look troubled,' said Mo.

'It is the fact that so many adults have ADHD but they have to deal with their own kids who have it too. It is so much work. I have to just concentrate on adults and older teenagers first, to get their lives into gear before I could ever concentrate on adults and kids together,' I replied.

'Which is a great start,' said Mo.

'I have to first start with me,' I said. 'But there is a huge worry, even after working so much ADHD stuff out which I cannot influence.'.

'What's that then?' asked Mo.

'I don't want to get to retirement age and the doctor doesn't prescribe me the medication anymore!'

'Why should that happen?' asked Mo.

'I just feel that ADHD is still not understood by so many people. There is a huge emphasis on prescribing the medication for people in employment, to do their jobs efficiently. All my prescribing doctor asks are questions about my job and if I have one or if it is going well. My medication is covered by my health insurance. When I don't work anymore, will it stop?'

'You don't know this,' said Mo.

'But I run an ADHD success group for people of all ages. When people cannot get their medications anymore, that's it. It's game over!'

'What do you mean?' asked Mo.

'You know what I mean, Mo.'

'Then people need to be self-sufficient,' said Mo.

'I agree, we cannot be tied into the job workplace. We have to find out where our strengths lie and make our own way in the world,'

Principles

- I knew that distractions in my environment were reduced significantly. What I was feeling for a long time was *myself.* This took me ten months to realise.
- Differentiate between impulsivity (which I don't have now) and being 'overly keen'.
- I started an hour of enjoyment with my kids instead of being a bystander when they did sport.
- I was started to win on the inside which attracted people to me.
- I make sure I check in with myself every hour of the day!
- I recognise that coming off the medication causes me to argue and say things I don't mean. Therefore, I actively take myself out of any environment where people are present to do guided meditation for an hour. Try this. Take responsibility. Find what works with you.
- But I will find that if I forget to meditate at the thirteen-hour point I always walk around for half an hour trying to find something, mostly my iPod for meditation. If my meds were working, I know where everything is. That's what the meds do! Perhaps you can see similarities? That is why I will keep as many things in order during the day so I can find things easily.
- When I re-enter my family environment, I am back to my cheery self.

Chapter Seventeen – At the end of the day

ADHD is what it is. A defect in the brain that doesn't allow the right chemicals to reach certain points in the brain. If you have ADHD, thinking you might have ADHD or are in the diagnosis phase and this book has given you a reason to think that something is different and fulfils certain knowledge and criteria that is useful to you, then I have fulfilled my role. People with ADHD make up but a small percentage of every community but as a world's total sum we are here in our droves. You will realise if you are diagnosed and take medication that you will see everything in your life differently. You step into a new puzzle. Reading and understanding a book for the first time is something I will never forget. Finishing jobs now gives me a sense of achievement. It could be possible for you to experience the same joy. You can most definitely improve your secure rating within yourself but be aware of your higher level of emotional attachment. Reducing this attachment by realising that a situation, meeting with someone is just a part of life rather than something more doesn't give you a feeling of split energy.

It is also very important to let relationships evolve. For a long time, I thought, Ok I have to mould myself to this environment like a chameleon who changed immediately. Relationships don't work that way. Slow is better. I couldn't learn the German language in a couple of weeks. This took years to master. So do relationships.

When undiagnosed you don't want to miss out on the next opportunity, the next moment, the information you hear from the teacher in a school environment. It is then impossible to work out which information is important and which isn't.

Bob Proctor (2015) talks about people in a general way, stating that,"The "Almosts`` are not lazy. Often they are busier than the very effective few. They putter around all day long and half the night, though they fail to accomplish anything of any real importance. They are held back by indecision, by a lack of organisation in their work, and by an overattention to minor details."(2015, P53/54).

When you have the diagnosis of ADHD and if you decided to use medication or use sport to help you, the distractions are gone. Lower the emotional element next. It makes a huge difference. Then use your strong emotional element in the areas of life that are important to you – relationships, social projects, your career (yes, you can have one now, even your own company!) or whatever you like.

Desire to learn and have the desire to drop old techniques that don't work.

Because I only have thirteen hours, I want to make the most of my time. The distraction comes back for me and millions of people every night. When the distraction in my life disappeared, I decided immediately not to do anything to deliberately shorten the rest of my life. John Maxwell once said "I am responsible to you, not for you."

I have two kids and it is difficult. I have to be responsible to and for them, like any parent, when they are young. It is easy to forget that we don't need the same approach in an adult world. People around you might not work as fast as you do. Take a step back sometimes. You may want to change everything at once, to finally get up to speed. Just don't rush.

Remember, it is not like you have climbed up a few steps within the last couple of days once you have been diagnosed. Expect people to leave you, even the ones you love. ADHD is a bit over the top for most people to handle. You just have to be happy with the new mission statement you design for yourself. I moved to southern Germany so my kids can have a richer childhood and I could finally get peace in my life.

As I sat down one night to write about an adventure, I had with the family that day I knew the first year of my new life with ADHD and medication had come to a close. I learnt a lot over this time. I later settled down with meditation and came face to face with Mo's image for the first time. He reached his hand out to mine and gave me a letter. It read:

Dear Simon,

I am glad you see me as a friendly voice. I have been with you every time you have picked up a pen to write those thousands of pages of notes over the years. They have really helped you, haven't they!

But I am glad I am here with you now. You let me out the box through your determination and your wife's help in suggesting going for an ADHD diagnosis. I know you are eternally grateful but I am glad you accepted me and don't take me for granted!

Writing your book has been a very tiring experience, trying to find the positives in life when you are subjected to a debilitating mental condition. But you didn't see it in this way. I could see you skilfully work your way through some real difficult life situations to grant you and others more understanding. But it is the silent skills that matter most. That's what I like about you, without being biased!

I want us to work together using a futuristic approach. Let your future pull you along. Do you know how good that feels? There is no fight anymore with something that isn't there.

I look forward to being your guide. I even look forward to helping you write the next thousands of notes you have in your head. I will be the one who decides which keys to press on the keyboard for your next book. I am you, you are me and I will never leave your side.

Love Mo.

I look up with tears streaming down my face. He was gone.

But I knew he would be back tomorrow.

References

Barkley, R.A. & Benton, C.M. (2010) *Taking Charge of Adult ADHD*. The Guildford Press.

Canfield, J. (2005) *How to Get from Where You Are to Where You Want to Be. The 25 Principles of Success*. Harper Collins Publishers Ltd.

Dienach, P A. Chronicles from the future. The amazing story of Paul Amadeus Dienach (2018), copyright Achulleas Sirigos. Edited by Achilleas Sirigos . This way out productions.

Fox, K. (2004) Watching the English. The Hidden Rules of English Behaviour. Hodder & Stoughton.

Hill, N. (2005) *Think and Grow Rich*. Penguin (originally published 1937).

Levine, A. & Rachel S.F Heller, R.S.F. (2010) *Attached*, Pan Macmillan.

Maxwell, J. (2011) *Winning is an Inside Job, The Power of Winning* [CD], Blackstone Audiobooks. 35:49–36:04.

Maxwell, J.C. (2016) *What Successful People Know About Leadership*.

Meyer, E. (2014) *The Culture Map*. Perseus Books Group.

Proctor, B. (2015) *The ABC's of Success – The Essential Principles from America's Greatest Prosperity Teacher*. Penguin.

Yung, C.G (1963) *Memories, Dreams, Reflections*. Pantheon.

Websites: For fitness – sharnyandjulius.com

The Big Thank you section.

When Dr Sophie Zötler (pediatrician) told me she wants the first copy of this book I knew I had to write it. She saw the value of the information and knew I could pull-it off. Thank you very much.

My ex-wife saw I had all of the traits of ADHD. Thank you very much for helping me to get a diagnosis.

I would like to thank my closest friends Chris Short, Caroline Seidig and Julia Voigt.

Last but not least, I would like to thank the Seattle Adults with ADHD Facebook site, especially Natalie Saxe for showing support of my book during the writing process.

www.ingramcontent.com/pod-product-compliance
Lightning Source LLC
Chambersburg PA
CBHW081201280526
45789CB00006B/2263